Wounded: Studies in Literary and Cinematic Trauma

Special Issue Editor

Gail Finney

MDPI • Basel • Beijing • Wuhan • Barcelona • Belgrade

MDPI

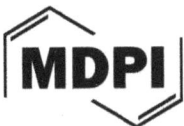

Special Issue Editor
Gail Finney
University of California
USA

Editorial Office
MDPI
St. Alban-Anlage 66
Basel, Switzerland

This edition is a reprint of the Special Issue published online in the open access journal *Humanities* (ISSN 2076-0787) from 2017–2018 (available at: http://www.mdpi.com/journal/humanities/special_issues/cinematic_trauma).

For citation purposes, cite each article independently as indicated on the article page online and as indicated below:

Lastname, F.M.; Lastname, F.M. Article title. *Journal Name* **Year**, *Article number*, page range.

First Editon 2018

Cover image courtesy of flickr user Porsche Brosseau.

ISBN 978-3-03842-935-7 (Pbk)
ISBN 978-3-03842-936-4 (PDF)

Table of Contents

About the Special Issue Editor

Gail Finney, Professor of Comparative Literature and German. Gail Finney was educated at Princeton University and the University of California, Berkeley. She taught formerly at Harvard University and is currently Professor of Comparative Literature and German at the University of California, Davis. Her publications include The Counterfeit Idyll: The Garden Ideal and Social Reality in Nineteenth-Century Fiction (1984), Women in Modern Drama: Freud, Feminism, and European Theater at the Turn of the Century (1989, 1991), Look Who's Laughing: Gender and Comedy (ed.) (1994), Christa Wolf (1999), Visual Culture in Twentieth-Century Germany: Text as Spectacle (ed.) (2006), "Ain güt geboren edel man": A Festschrift for Winder McConnell on the Occasion of his Sixty-fifth Birthday (coed.) (2011), Literature of Fantasy and the Supernatural (ed.) (2012, 2013), and numerous articles on 19th-and 20th-century German and comparative literature.

Preface to "Wounded: Studies in Literary and Cinematic Trauma"

We live in an era of traumatic discourse. The wound (trauma is the Greek word for "wound") speaks multiple languages. Often, the trauma registered is political—the trauma of war in Syria, Afghanistan, Iraq, and other nations and the concomitant European migrant crisis. Literature and films about Hiroshima, Vietnam, the "Dirty War" in Argentina, 9/11, and, perhaps above all, the Holocaust, abound. We encounter memoirs of survivors and memoirs of the children of survivors, in connection with whom Marianne Hirsch has coined the term "postmemory." Furthermore, the recent series of brutal and unjust actions toward unarmed blacks by white law officers is generating a new discourse of the long-standing trauma of race relations in the United States.

Autobiographical and other narratives of family trauma are also flourishing. Memoirs by the dozen seek to come to terms with childhood and youthful experiences scarred by radical alienation between family members, extreme poverty, addictions of all kinds, child and spousal abuse, child molestation, parent–child incest, sibling incest, divorce, suicide, and murder.

The traumatic experience is frequently rendered in fantastic terms, as in the manifold science fiction and horror representations of vampires, zombies, ghosts, and interstellar travelers, which can be read as displaced manifestations of post-9/11 paranoia or of a generalized culture of trauma.

The eleven articles in this volume employ a variety of interpretive approaches to collective or individual trauma as depicted in literature and films. The cultures of ancient Greece, Germany, Argentina, the United States, France, and Chile are represented.

Gail Finney
Special Issue Editor

![humanities logo] *humanities*

MDPI

Article

One Voice Too Many: Echoes of Irony and Trauma in *Oedipus the King*

Joshua Waggoner

Department of English, University of Tampa, Tampa, FL 33606, USA; jwaggoner@ut.edu

Academic Editor: Gail Finney

Received: 30 September 2017; Accepted: 3 November 2017; Published: 9 November 2017

Abstract: Sophocles' *Oedipus the King* has often inspired concurrent interpretations examining the tragic irony of the play and the traumatic neurosis of its protagonist. The Theban king epitomizes a man who knows everything but himself, and Sophocles' use of irony allows Oedipus to discover the truth in a manner that Freud viewed in *The Interpretation of Dreams* as "comparable to the work of a psychoanalysis." Psychoanalytical readings of Oedipus at times depend greatly on his role as a doubled figure, but this article specifically investigates his doubled voice in order to demonstrate the interrelated, chiasmic relationship between Oedipus' trauma and the trope of irony. It argues, in fact, that irony serves as the language, so to speak, of the traumatic experiences haunting the king and his city, but it also posits that this doubled voice compounds the irony of the play and its hero. In other words, in addition to the Sophoclean irony that dominates the work, the doubling of the king's voice reveals a modified form of Socratic irony that contributes to the tragedy's power. Consequently, even after the king's recognition of the truth ultimately resolves the work's tragic irony, Oedipus remains divided by a state of simultaneous knowledge and ignorance.

Keywords: Oedipus; trauma; neurosis; irony; voice; doubled; echo; knowledge; ignorance

---

> For there are in the play not one Oedipus but two.
>
> —Bernard Knox

According to Friedrich Hölderlin's diagnosis, the Theban king suffers from a problem of sight: "Perhaps King Oedipus had an eye too many" (Hölderlin 1984, p. 253). He possesses too much insight and subsequently seeks out knowledge beyond the scope of what is necessary or prudent. Hölderlin argues that Oedipus encounters trouble when he "*interprets* the oracle *too infinitely*" by linking together, with some assistance from Creon, Apollo's commandment to purge the city of corruption with the murder of Laius, the former king of Thebes (Hölderlin 1986, pp. 232–33). His capacity for unravelling riddles, which proved so valuable before the Sphinx, now imbues Oedipus with the confidence that his interpretation of the Oracle is the right one, and in the end we discover that this confidence is well founded. The king is correct once again, but Hölderlin claims that such knowledge has an intoxicating and dangerous effect that "provokes itself to know more than it can bear or grasp" (Hölderlin 1986, p. 233). His eyes, in a sense, are bigger than his stomach.

Nevertheless, Hölderlin's reference to the king's additional eye in his poem "In lieblicher Bläu" ('In Lovely Blue') immediately transitions in the following line from a problem of vision to a problem of voice: "This / man's suffering seems indescribable, unspeakable, / inexpressible" (Hölderlin 1984, p. 253). Although Hölderlin believes that what Oedipus discovers with his vaunted insight is ineffable in nature, there is an alternate reading of *Oedipus the King* that depends not upon the king having no voice but rather upon him having one voice too many. In the same way that Hölderlin attributes to Oedipus a superfluous eye that extends his interpretive powers past their limits, the king is also afflicted with a doubled voice that multiplies what we might consider the story of Oedipus, thereby obscuring and fragmenting his identity. If it is Oedipus' extra eye that allows him to discover truths he cannot bear, it is the echo of his own voice that renders those truths unbearable.

In a particular sense, Hölderlin's interpretation echoes Tiresias's attempt, early in the play, to warn Oedipus and the audience of this doubled voice, a warning that also switches from vision to speech. The seer's diagnosis of the king begins with the same play on sight and knowledge that Sophocles consistently weaves throughout the tragedy:

> "The double lash of your mother and your father's curse / will whip you from this land one day, their footfall / treading you down in terror, darkness shrouding / your eyes that can now see the light!"

But in the subsequent lines Tiresias shifts directly from Oedipus' future blindness to questions regarding the doubling of his voice:

> Soon, soon
> You'll scream aloud—what haven won't reverberate?
> What rock of Cithaeron won't scream back in echo?
> That day you learn the truth about your marriage,
> the wedding-march that sang you into your halls,
> the lusty voyage home to the fatal harbor!

(Sophocles 1984, ll. 476–84)[1]

Through his prophecy, Tiresias locates the origin of this additional voice in the rocks of Cithaeron, which reverberate with Oedipus' cries. By conjoining the king's voice[s] with the mountains outside Thebes, the prophet acknowledges the trauma at the play's heart, which splits Oedipus' identity and creates his doubled voice. In other words, Sophocles does not construct *Oedipus the King* around a story that is ineffable or inexpressible but rather around a story rendered ambiguous by the irony of its language and circumstance and the traumatized fragmentation of its hero. Oedipus' doubled voice tells two stories and he is the author of both, but the king does not recognize or recall the true narrative until the two voices are rejoined.

The result of this twofold voice is what Maurice Blanchot calls a "silent dialogue," in which Oedipus converses "with the silence of the gods—the speech of the solitary man, a speech in itself divided and truly cut in two because of the silent sky with which it pursues its invincible discourse" (Blanchot 1997, p. 201). Oedipus receives no justification from the gods for his terrible fate, but Blanchot considers this heavenly silence to be productive in that the lack of a response provides a particular kind of answer, even if in the negative. Oedipus' compulsion to fill the emptiness caused by the missing response provokes a self-reflexivity that leads to epiphany. It creates, in other words, a psychological division in the Theban king that leads eventually to self-knowledge and the rediscovery of a trauma that is already inherently divided between knowing and not knowing. All the while, the conduit for this discovery is Oedipus' compounded voice, which proves to be as symptomatic as it is revelatory of his traumatic origin and identity.

The split is already spelled out in the name of Oedipus. The riddle regarding how to decipher the root "oid-" has long caused interpretative problems for the play's characters and its critics. "Οἶδα, the knowledge of the *tyrannos*, ποὺσ, the swollen foot of Laius' son—in the hero's name the basic equation is already symbolically present, the equation which Oedipus will finally solve," Bernard Knox writes of this ambiguity (Knox 1979, p. 100) but this almost glides too smoothly over the trouble in the first half of the equation because "Oid-" can signify both 'knowledge' and 'swollen.' The characters make their own critical decisions about how to read the significance of the name, decisions that betray their particular perspectives, and Pietro Pucci notes that it is often the 'swollen'

---

[1] All citations and translations are from Robert Fagles's version of *Oedipus the King* with accompanying line number.

foot that is forgotten: "The text intimates by parechesis the connection of 'Oidipous' with the verb *oida* ('I know') and writes off the meaning that has in fact been at the origin of his name, from *oidao*, *oideo*, ('to become swollen') and accordingly, 'Swollenfoot'" (Pucci 1988, p. 149). Because the play begins after Oedipus has already won his reputation for wisdom and riddle-solving, the 'oida/I know' root becomes the dominant reading. In the priest's opening plea, for example, he praises the intelligence that saved Thebes from the Sphinx and reveals the city's investment in the 'know' etymology. After all, their salvation relies upon this reading of the king's name, and they are justified in the end, despite the catastrophic effect Oedipus' knowledge brings down upon his own head.

It does not take long, of course, for Oedipus to fully adopt the more flattering nickname. Perhaps too willingly, he emphasizes this version of his name in his confrontation with Tiresias: "But I came by, Oedipus the ignorant, / I stopped the Sphinx! With no help from the birds, / the flight of my own intelligence hit the mark" (ll. 451–53). Pucci uses the parechesis of the line *'ho meden eidos Oidipous'* to argue that, "its sarcastic innuendo suggests that Oedipus reads his name as 'Know...'" (Pucci 1988, p. 150). The outburst therefore represents an unusual break from the play's dominant Sophoclean irony as Oedipus mixes hubris and Socratic irony in order to elide the connection between his name and his limp. His remark, in other words, betrays an attempt to forget an earlier wound. Like the priest before him, the interpretive urge toward 'I know' and away from 'swollen' helps to cement Oedipus' political position because, as Knox explains, "his knowledge is what makes him *tyrannos*, confident and decisive; knowledge has made man what he is, master of the world" (Knox 1979, p. 100). Nevertheless, Sophocles' mastery of tragic irony, which reveals the gap between the character's ignorance and the listener's knowledge, never allows the audience to feel comfortable with the king's reading of his own name.

In Oedipus' epithet, the convergence of this Sophoclean irony and the Socratic irony in which the king 'pretends' to be ignorant creates a knot of simultaneously valid and oppositional meanings that quickly exceed the king's ability to control them. His feigned self-deprecation slips from his grasp and reopens an old wound instead of damaging the blind seer at whom it was aimed. Cynthia Chase analyzes the blowback Oedipus experiences from his attempted sarcasm:

> In the very act of claiming reasoned control over language, Oedipus utters
> syllables that speak the opposite; the controlling utterance here is not his,
> but that of a fragmentary language speaking itself. "Lack- knowing- I know-
> foot": in the very act of deploying a limited local irony, with his sarcastic
> references to himself as "the ignorant," Oedipus produces an irony of that irony,
> which fragments meaning into material signifiers.
>
> (Chase 1979, p. 61)

Chase isolates the way in which the tragic irony of the play manages to preserve the literal meaning of 'ignorant' despite Oedipus' ironic intention; he unwittingly hits upon the truth of his situation, or he allows the audience to do so at the least. Even so, once one recognizes the uncontrollable play of the language, the ambiguity of the line begins to multiply until it escapes the grasp of the audience just as it had previously escaped Oedipus. For Chase, this is a purposeful mechanism designed to make the audience forget (momentarily) their complicity with Oedipus. "The double meanings thus mark our distance only to draw us in," she writes (Chase 1979, p. 62). For my purposes, however, both Pucci and Chase have relied too heavily on the connection of Oedipus' name with the root *oida* ('I know'). Taking into consideration the fact that the more appropriate linguistic connotation resides with *oidao* ("to become swollen") (Pucci 1988, p. 149), the possible significations of the line double again after reintroducing the original root:

1. Lack- knowing- I know- foot (literal) → Ignorant Oedipus
2. Lack- knowing- I know- foot (ironic) → Knowledgeable Oedipus
3. Lack- knowing- swollen- foot (literal) → Ignorant Oedipus
4. Lack- knowing- swollen- foot (ironic) → Knowledgeable Oedipus

Employing what Chase calls the 'limited local irony' of sarcasm, Oedipus seems to mean the second sense, but the tragic irony of the plot disrupts his intention and causes the second meaning to collapse back into the first: Oedipus is actually ignorant. While this reading of the line is entirely valid and appropriate, the substitution of *oida* with *oideo/oidao* is ultimately more significant because it produces an irony (present in the fourth sense of the line) that more aptly represents the doubling that Oedipus undergoes during the traumatic moments that instigate the tragedy's action.

Although it may appear at first that the second and fourth interpretations of the line "ὁ μηδὲν εἰδὼσ Οἰδίπουσ" contain negligible differences, the transition between 'Know-Foot' and 'Swollen-Foot' significantly alters the referent of the knowledgeable version of Oedipus. The interpretive knot grows more entangled as new questions arise. In addition to *whether* Oedipus knows or does not know, it becomes less clear *what* he knows and even more importantly, the line also obscures *who* it is that does the knowing. In terms of the second construction (Oedipus' intended meaning), 'I know' refers specifically to the solution of the Sphinx's riddle, which liberates Thebes and places Oedipus on the throne. On the other hand, as Chase explains, once his irony collapses back on him, the referent changes to the trauma of his origins as Oedipus shifts from knowledge to ignorance; his statement proves true rather than sarcastic. However, when *oida* becomes *oideo / oidao* in the third and fourth constructions, the line both retains and revises Chase's referent in the sense that the thing known remains the traumatic event but the person who possesses the knowledge transforms from 'Know-Foot' to 'Swollen-Foot.' This is where the chaos of the play's irony becomes most bewildering because 'Know-Foot' now represents a version of Oedipus that is ignorant and 'Swollen-Foot' embodies one who has known all along, who possesses knowledge of an event the significance of which has yet to be discovered. As a result, the play generates much of its power from a kind of chiasmic interplay between irony and trauma, in which the latter produces a fissure (in terms of knowledge) that then creates a space in which the former can function (in terms of language).

This leads us back again to the doubled nature of Oedipus' psyche, which results from the traumatic series of events in which he is abandoned by his parents and subsequently murders one and procreates with the other. Knox describes this doubling in terms of a psychological game of cat-and-mouse:

> One [Oedipus] is the magnificent figure set before us in the opening scenes, *tyrannos*, the man of wealth and power, first of men, the intellect and energy which drive on the search. The other is the object of the search, a shadowy figure who has violated the most fundamental human taboos, an incestuous parricide, "most accursed of men."

> (Knox 1979, p. 99)

Here Knox distinguishes the perpetrator from the king, but he also recognizes that these two figures occupy the same space, adding, "And even before the one Oedipus finds the other, they are connected and equated in the name which they both bear, Oedipus" (Knox 1979, p. 99). On the other hand, the malleable nature at the root of *Oidipous* means that the name of the king and the name of the parricide are not precisely the same. At the moment of his transgression, Oedipus can only be named 'Swollen-Foot' because he has not yet earned the reputation behind his 'Know-Foot' nickname. Likewise, within the action of the play, Oedipus avoids acknowledging his 'Swollen-Foot' name because he has repressed the traumatic events that occurred while bearing it. The king addresses this possibility only in his discussion with the messenger, who recognizes him as the infant with the bound feet. Regarding the 'Swollen-Foot' name, Pucci notes that "this etymology is, so to speak, the inscription on his feet that both functions as a recognition sign and agrees with the oracular inscription" (Pucci 1988, p. 149). The timing is significant because the acknowledgement of the *oideo / oidao* root coincides with the revelation that Oedipus is not Polybus' son, thereby marking the early limits of Oedipus' recognition and the moment at which his 'old affliction' begins to come to light (Sophocles 1984, l. 1132). Sophocles uses the reappearance of 'Swollen-Foot' to catalyse the king's return to the traumas of his youth; like the hysterical patients Sigmund Freud would study so many years later, Oedipus begins to "suffer mostly from reminiscences" (Breuer and Freud 1961, p. 4). He begins to remember experiences that he has forgotten but has always in some sense known.

By 1920, Freud's theory of 'reminiscences' had evolved into the 'compulsion to repeat' (especially strong in traumatized patients) found in *Beyond the Pleasure Principle*. The patient, Freud writes, "is obliged to *repeat* the repressed material as a contemporary experience instead of, as the physician would prefer to see, *remembering* it as something belonging to the past" (Freud 1961, p. 19). The unique case of Oedipus, however, is more complex because he acts as both patient and physician. The over-confident investigator ('Know-Foot') is determined to discover a past that he ('Swollen-Foot') is simultaneously desperate to repress, and the irony of this internal conflict is that 'Know-Foot' remains in the dark while 'Swollen-Foot' clings to the shadows precisely because he is privy to the truth. The former represents the man who has saved Thebes and seeks to do so again. The latter, meanwhile, has been lost in the incomplete experience of the traumatic event and now must be exposed, rediscovered, punished.

The relationship between these two versions of Oedipus is most evident in Freud's later discussion, in *Moses and Monotheism*, of the twofold effect of trauma on the psyche. Positive reactions to the trauma constitute "endeavors to revive the trauma, to remember the forgotten experience, or, better still, to make it real—to live through once more a repetition of it" (Freud 1939, p. 95). This urge clearly dominates the 'Know-Foot' Oedipus, who is relentless in his pursuit of the truth. His 'fixation to the trauma,' as Freud labels it, will not allow him to stop his ears, but it also encounters opposition from the negative effect of trauma, which struggles against repetition: "The negative reactions pursue the opposite aim; here nothing is to be remembered or repeated of the forgotten traumata. They may be grouped together as defensive reactions. They express themselves in avoiding issues, a tendency which may culminate in an inhibition or phobia" (Freud 1939, p. 95). This avoidance of the issue has been the function of the 'Swollen-Foot' Oedipus ever since the traumas of his infancy and youth and for many years the defensive reaction was stunningly successful. Through the riddle of the Sphinx, the acquisition of a kingdom, the marriage to a queen and the birth of four children, 'Swollen-Foot' remains locked in the depths of Oedipus' psyche, refusing either remembrance or resolution. Only after the devastation of the blight and the oracle's command to drive pollution from the land does Oedipus unwittingly turn his riddle-solving prowess inward and the truth of his experience subsequently starts to surface.

At first the process is slow and arduous. A random memory flashes as Jocasta tells the story of her first husband's death: "Strange, hearing you just now," Oedipus confesses, "my mind wandered, my thoughts racing back and forth" (Sophocles 1984, ll. 800–2). With each clue, 'Know-Foot' descends deeper into his unconscious, but the further he descends, the more 'Swollen-Foot' resists, constructing the inhibitions and phobias that must be overcome. "But my mother's bed, surely I must fear—" Oedipus reasons after he realizes only half the prophecy has been disproven (l. 1068), and later, when the herdsman warns, "Oh no, I'm right at the edge, the horrible truth—I've got to say it!" Oedipus rails, "And I'm at the edge of hearing horrors, yes, but I must hear!" (ll. 1283–85). Even 'Swollen-Foot's' attempt to resist "hearing horrors" is countermanded by 'Know-Foot's' insistence that he continue to listen. The give and take between the two figures is characteristic of the neurotic symptoms that "constitute a compromise, to which both the positive and negative effects of the trauma contribute; sometimes one component, sometimes the other, predominates. These opposite reactions create conflicts which the subject cannot as a rule resolve" (Freud 1939, p. 96). And so Sophocles' play, by beginning after the traumatic events have passed, revolves around the conflict between two versions or divisions of its tragic hero.

This framing of the play's action is what prompts Freud, in *The Interpretation of Dreams*, to note that *Oedipus the King* is "comparable to the work of a psychoanalysis" (Freud 1940, p. 160). Chase's analysis of this remark makes the connection more explicit by arguing that, "*Oedipus Tyrannus* successfully dramatizes the activity of repression and unrepression—the 'abnormal defense' that characterizes 'psychoneurosis' and the peculiar 'process of revealing' that constitutes interpretation of dreams, or psychoanalysis" (Chase 1979, pp. 56–57). Because Chase focuses on Freud and not Sophocles, however, her essay declines to explore the specific literary methods by which Sophocles 'successfully dramatizes' these activities, methods which rely significantly on the figure of the voice and the trope of irony.

The Voices of Oedipus

Multiple times throughout *Oedipus the King*, Sophocles invokes the figure of the disembodied voice to speak to the 'Know-Foot' Oedipus. At times, this voice will serve to warn Oedipus about the dangers lurking in the truth he seeks, while at others it represents a truth that he should and in some ways does already know, but in each instance Sophocles leaves the speaker ambiguous. It seems to me, however, that the disembodied voice betrays its own origin, speaking out from the 'Swollen-Foot' version of the king, and its resonance becomes both a symptom and a representation of Oedipus' original traumatization.

Jocasta, for example, recognizes the danger of this disembodied or unconscious voice, although she misidentifies what is dangerous about it. Speaking to the chorus, she laments her inability to prevent her anxious husband from listening. She notes that her husband is "beside himself" and complains that, "he's at the mercy of every passing voice, if the voice tells of terror" (ll. 1001, 1004–5). The queen purposefully resorts to a vague, disconnected voice because she wants to emphasize its fleeting nature, its lack of foundation in the sense of both locus and truth. Following the pattern of the play, however, Jocasta says more than she means as tragic irony compounds the significance of the lines. The audience knows that the 'passing voice,' which echoes warnings from the Oracle and Tiresias, specifically seeks to communicate what are, from the perspective of 'Swollen-Foot,' the terrible ramifications of his traumatic past. The queen attempts to minimize this terror because she has no desire to listen to the voice, but Oedipus feels compelled to hear because he suffers from a neurosis that Freud sees "as a direct expression of a 'fixation' to an early period of their past" (Freud 1939, p. 96). Jocasta therefore unwittingly describes the symptomatic compulsiveness that results from the internal antagonism between her husband's positive and negative reactions to trauma, which are together expressed through a doubled voice.

Unsurprisingly, the first instance of this voice is heard by the seer, Tiresias, who with characteristic prescience identifies it before it has spoken. Returning again to the scene in which he angrily interrogates the king about his parentage, we see the prophet adopt his own brand of Socratic irony by asking a question to which he already knows the answer: "Soon, soon / you'll scream aloud—what haven won't reverberate? What rock of Cithaeron won't scream back in echo?" (ll. 479–81). Tiresias doubles the voice in an echo that rebounds back on Oedipus because the power of the prophecy exists not in the scream itself but rather in the place from which it is repeated: the rock of Cithaeron. Thomas Gould explicitly marks the importance of this line, explaining that Cithaeron is "a very special mountain: it is where Oedipus was exposed as a child, and where he will beg to be exiled to when he has blinded himself. Teiresias and the audience know this, but Oedipus and the Chorus do not" (Gould 1970, p. 66, n. 421). In other words, the doubled voice functions as a trigger for the prophecy's tragic irony, but there is an additional, secondary consequence of the echo and its geographical origin. Tiresias's specific mention of the mountain on which the infant Oedipus was exposed allows us to read one voice (the scream) as originating from 'Know-Foot' Oedipus while a second voice (the echo) reverberates from 'Swollen-Foot' Oedipus, who already knows, like the prophet, the trauma that prompts the cries and has the wounds to prove it. Later in the play, the voice will again emanate from precisely these wounds.

After the messenger arrives at Thebes to spread the news of Polybus' death, he attempts to assuage the king's anxiety by proving that Polybus and Merope are not Oedipus' biological parents. He relates the story of rescuing Oedipus at Cithaeron and then, when Oedipus asks why he needed rescue, the messenger responds as though the king should already be aware of his history: "Your ankles ... they tell the story. Look at them" (l. 1131). He describes how the king's feet were fettered and adds, "you got your name from that misfortune too, the name's still with you" (ll. 1135–36). For corroboration, the messenger effectively disowns his claim to the story by explaining that the wounds in Oedipus' feet have already told the tale. In this instance, the voice comes from the literal 'Swollen-Foot' at the root of Oedipus' name and then expands out to the figurative 'Swollen-Foot' existing within Oedipus' psyche. Again, the (partially) disembodied voice resonates from a locus that already knows the story of the trauma.

At this point, because the discussion consists of the witnessing and representation of a trauma, one cannot avoid its similarity to Cathy Caruth's theory of trauma, which likewise focuses on a wound that speaks. In order to explore the ramifications of a wound that bears witness, Caruth reinterprets Freud's allusion in *Beyond the Pleasure Principle* not to Sophocles' Oedipus but rather to Torquato Tasso's Tancred and Clorinda.[2] Caruth claims that the strength of the scene lies not only in the *repetition* of a wound but also (and perhaps more so) in "the moving and sorrowful *voice* that cries out, a voice that is paradoxically released *through the wound*." She continues:

> The voice of [Tancred's] beloved addresses him and, in this address, bears
> witness to the past he has unwittingly repeated. Tancred's story thus repre-
> sents traumatic experience not only as the enigma of a human agent's
> repeated and unknowing acts but also as the enigma of the otherness of a
> human voice that cries out from the wound, a voice that witnesses a truth
> that Tancred himself cannot fully know.
>
> (Caruth 1996, pp. 2–3)

With a few alterations, this argument could fit Oedipus and his wounded ankles as smoothly as it does Tancred and Clorinda. Indeed Caruth proposes for Tancred something analogous to the 'Know-Foot'/'Swollen-Foot' relationship that exists within Oedipus. Despite the fact that her emphasis is on the voice of the other, she never closes off the possibility of understanding "the voice of Clorinda, within the parable of the example, to represent the other within the self that retains the memory of the 'unwitting' traumatic events of one's past" (Caruth 1996, p. 8). In this interpretation, the words that spill out of the wound represent Tancred's own voice rising up from the unconscious and taking the form of the positive, psychoneurotic, "compulsion to repeat."[3] For Oedipus, a similar and undeniable repetition compulsion forces to the surface the repressed voice within him. 'Swollen-Foot' speaks through his ankle wounds in order to warn 'Know-Foot' of the trauma at the core of his origin, a trauma that 'Know-Foot' does not fully know and which he therefore insists be raked up, heard, brought to light.

This means that Freud, if he desired, could easily have substituted the allusion to Tasso's poem by returning once again to the oedipal well for an illustration of his psychoanalytical theory. The wounds marking Oedipus' feet reveal an earlier manifestation of the psychological trouble

---

2   Freud refers to the episode in books 12 and 13 of *Gerusalemme Liberata* in which "Its hero, Tancred, unwittingly kills his beloved Clorinda in a duel while she is disguised in the armor of an enemy knight. After her burial he makes his way into a strange magic forest which strikes the Crusaders' army with terror. He slashes with his sword at a tall tree; but blood streams from the cut and the voice of Clorinda, whose soul is imprisoned in the tree, is heard complaining that he has wounded his beloved once again" (Freud 1961, p. 24).

3   Caruth eventually moves away from this reading of Tancred's voice because, as with Chase's reading of *Oedipus*, she is invested in demonstrating that Tancred's story is "the story of psychoanalytic writing itself" (Caruth 1996, pp. 8–9). Such a movement requires the voice of Clorinda to come from *outside* Tancred; nevertheless, Caruth never claims that these readings are mutually exclusive.

Tancred encounters in the forest outside Jerusalem. Both represent an event that is experienced without being fully understood and so Oedipus suffers from a trauma that exists not only in his past but also "in the way that its very unassimilated nature—the way it was precisely *not known* in the first instance—returns to haunt the survivor later on" (Caruth 1996, p. 4). In the case of King Oedipus, however, it would be incorrect to say that the circumstances of the past are 'not known.' He perhaps lacks *full* comprehension, which Caruth hints at above, but something else is at work in the play that renders Oedipus simultaneously knowledgeable and ignorant. The experience of trauma creates an internal conflict that doubles Oedipus, both in wound and voice, and Sophocles represents the conflict by means of a doubled ironic mode. The first, most commonly identified form is the tragic irony of the play itself and the second, more hidden and obscured form is a modified type of Socratic irony exhibited within Oedipus.

One of the most remarkable effects of the irony Sophocles employs throughout *Oedipus the King* is the way it represents the division Oedipus endures on account of his traumatic neurosis. Irony acts, in a sense, as the language of trauma and so Oedipus' doubled voice constitutes both a symptom and a cause of the neurosis. Jean-Pierre Vernant appears, in fact, to be working toward this effect of the play's irony when he argues that, "the ambiguity of [Oedipus'] words translates not the duplicity of his character, which is all of a piece, but more profoundly the duality of his being. Oedipus is double . . . Oedipus does not hear the secret discourse which is established, without his knowing it, at the heart of his own discourse" (Vernant 1978, p. 477), except that, in my view, Oedipus *does know*, at least in part, the secret at the heart of the play because this knowledge is the consequence of traumatic neurosis and the repression of his experience.

To reiterate, we know that Freud recognized *Oedipus the King* to be "comparable to the work of psychoanalysis" primarily because of the delayed discovery of the king's true identity (Freud 1940, p. 160). The correlation is made possible in part by the play's tragic irony, which transforms the audience and certain characters (i.e., Tiresias and the shepherd) into the analyst who watches the analysand (Oedipus) come to terms with his past. Nevertheless, the fact that Oedipus represents both investigator and perpetrator complicates this analogy because it means that he also functions to some extent as both analyst and analysand. Consequently, in order for the Oedipus that we have been calling 'Know-Foot' to successfully draw the truth from the Oedipus known as 'Swollen-Foot,' he must employ a complex, altered form of Socratic irony in which he pretends that he does not know the truth.

The objection at this point is that Socratic irony cannot be present within Oedipus because he is not pretending when he behaves as though he is ignorant of his past. Such an interpretation of the play is defensible, of course, but Oedipus' characteristic traumatic neurosis contributes another layer to the story that makes the opposite argument equally valid. Put another way, because we are dealing with trauma rather than run-of-the-mill ignorance or even fate, Oedipus as a doubled figure with a doubled voice exists on both planes; he both knows and does not know. It may be the case in fact that this separation and simultaneity is precisely what allows Oedipus and the play to reach their ultimate conclusion. *Oedipus the King* is like witnessing the psychoanalysis of a patient because, as Freud tells us, the treatment "must get him to re-experience some portion of his forgotten life, but must see to it, on the other hand, that the patient *retains some degree of aloofness*, which will enable him, in spite of everything, to recognize that what appears to be reality is in fact only a reflection of a forgotten past" (Freud 1961, p. 19, italics mine). The 'aloofness' necessary to the treatment represents a different term for what one might view as the irony of the play and its tragic hero. Oedipus is both ignorant of his past (Sophoclean irony) and unconsciously aware of it (Socratic irony) because of a faulty assimilation of its traumatic nature.

I recognize that an argument for Socratic irony in *Oedipus the King* might seem excessive and unnecessary considering the work that tragic irony does throughout, but my claim is that there is something extraordinary or idiosyncratic about the case of Oedipus that makes both types of irony necessary to cover the complexity of the play. There are several ways, in fact, that Oedipus acts as an outlier that resist some of the most famous elements of the tragedy. For example, Chase points out that Oedipus is paradoxically the only human to lack an Oedipus complex because his motives are not based on desire: "The one person who actually enacts patricide and incest completely misses the experience—until after the fact, when the parrincest is inscribed as a palimpsest and becomes readable for the first time" (Chase 1979, p. 58). Additionally, the missed experience of this 'parrincest' is made possible in part by his solution of the Sphinx's riddle, but the answer he gives does not fully apply to him. In its formulation from Apollodorus' *Library*, the riddle asks, "What is that which has one voice and yet becomes four-footed and two-footed and three-footed?" (Rokem 1996, p. 257). And yet, as we have seen, Oedipus' voice is doubled. He does not have 'one voice,' which means he does not conform neatly to the category of 'mankind' constituting the riddle's solution. Oedipus' exceptional identity often exceeds the categories existing in and produced by the play and so the general application of tragic irony to Sophocles' protagonist encounters similar resistance because his traumatic neurosis complicates the type of knowledge differential consistent with the trope.

This is not at all to say that Oedipus does not participate in the tragic irony of Sophocles' tragedy. In fact, if one thinks of Kenneth Burke's definition of "true irony," which "is based upon a sense of fundamental kinship with the enemy, as one *needs* him, is *indebted* to him, is not merely outside him as an observer but contains him *within*, being consubstantial with him" (Burke 1941, p. 435), then Oedipus epitomizes the trope since he embodies both 'Know-Foot' and 'Swollen-Foot.' The oppositional pair located within the king makes the tragic irony of the play possible, but it also calls attention to the traumatic neurosis, which, as Michael Lambek suggests, "might be redescribed as being sick in an ironic mode" (Lambek 2003, p. 14). In other words, there is a correlation between the trope and the neurosis that emerges most significantly in the character of Oedipus.

Paul Antze, who has investigated this connection from an anthropological perspective, confirms the link between the *Oedipus the King* and psychoanalysis by arguing that a patient suffering the throes of neurosis will, like the Theban king, seek out the answer through psychoanalytical treatment. When confronted, however, by the tragic irony that he is the source of his own trouble, "the patient's behavior begins to take on the kind of ironic doubleness found in *Oedipus Rex*, in which the protagonist's very denials somehow affirm what he denies" (Antze 2003, p. 117). Yet Antze's use of the general term 'somehow' is not quite appropriate in this case. Because we are dealing with a king (and a patient) who suffers from traumatic neurosis, the source of the affirmations that refute his denials is neither mysterious nor unknown. In truth, the affirmations originate from the 'Swollen-Foot' figure who "knew it all along," so to speak, and this internal knowledge creates resistance for interpreting Oedipus as ironic in a purely tragic or Sophoclean sense.

Because Oedipus is not strictly ignorant of his circumstances, the knowledge differential exhibited by the king breaks through the standard conception of tragic irony and crosses over into the modified form of Socratic irony that we have been progressing toward, in which he divides himself between one who knows and one who does not. Antze also explores the possible role of Socratic irony in neurotic behavior, writing that:

> Because of their ambiguity, neurotic symptoms also lend themselves to the kind
> of covert commentary we associate with irony—allowing the sufferer to express
> feelings in a way that escapes repercussions . . . The one difference, albeit a
> crucial one, is that the neurotic doesn't "know" what she is doing. The gap
> between knowledge and ignorance that makes irony possible appears here as a
> gap between conscious and unconscious knowledge.

(Antze 2003, p. 114)

Conscious and unconscious knowledge is precisely the complicating factor in the case of Oedipus. In psychoanalytical terms, the feigned ignorance of the *Eirôn* becomes the repressed knowledge of the neurotic; the internal conflict waged within Oedipus plays itself out like a singular dialectic or Blanchot's 'solitary dialogue.' One voice speaks and another voice answers within the same identity.

It is the relationship between knowledge and ignorance that marks both Oedipus' neurosis and the play's irony, but the Theban king is not ignorant enough to participate fully in Sophoclean irony and he lacks the conscious knowledge to participate fully in Socratic irony. In each instance he is too large for the category and so he straddles the borders, standing with a foot in each. The tension of this position provides the tension of the play as the 'Know-Foot' and the 'Swollen-Foot' figures clash and corrupt each other. "To that wise, knowing master of Thebes, whom happy omen protects, is at every point opposed the cursed infant, the Swollen Foot cast out of his fatherland," writes Vernant, "But in order for Oedipus really to know who he is, the first of the two characters which he initially assumed must be inverted until it turns into the second" (Vernant 1978, p. 483). 'Know-Foot' must cede his power and position to 'Swollen-Foot,' which he does after [re]learning the truth of his identity from the herdsman: "O god— / all come true, all burst to light! / O light—now let me look my last on you! / I stand revealed at last— / cursed in my birth, cursed in marriage, / cursed in the lives I cut down with these hands!" (ll. 1305–10).

In his *Poetics*, Aristotle believes that this moment of simultaneous recognition (*anagnorisis*) and reversal (*peripeteia*), in which the former leads directly to the latter, makes Oedipus' the best of all tragic recognitions (Aristotle 1997, p. 72). There is a sense, however, that this recognition and reversal resolves only half the story because, while the tragic irony dissipates as the truth comes to light, Oedipus retains much of the Socratic irony that had previously been overshadowed by its Sophoclean counterpart.

In the end, with Jocasta hanged and Oedipus blinded, Sophocles includes another figure of the disembodied or doubled voice, one that hints at a remainder left over after the convergence of 'Know-Foot' and 'Swollen-Foot.' Before the chorus, Oedipus cries out: "Oh, Ohh— / the agony! I am agony— / where am I going? where on earth? / where does all this agony hurl me? / where's my voice?— / winging, swept away on a dark tide—" (ll. 1442–47). The scene is remarkable because, at the very moment in the tragedy when Oedipus is supposed to have closed the gap in his knowledge and discovered the truth of his circumstances, he is left with nothing but questions and one of these questions is particularly puzzling: "Where is my voice? winging, swept away on a dark tide" (ll. 1446-47). Throughout the play, the 'Know-Foot' version of Oedipus felt confident that all the prophecies were incorrect because the shepherd, the only living witness to Laius's death, had testified that *several* highwaymen were responsible for the murder. "If he still holds to the same number," Oedipus remarks to Jocasta, "I cannot be the killer. One can't equal many" (ll. 933–34). Nevertheless, the effect of Oedipus' traumatic neurosis is that he *can* equal many and he does so in the doubled form of his name and voice. As a result, when he asks where his voice is "winging, swept away on a dark tide" (l. 1447), he is not only questioning where into the darkness before him his voice has gone. He is also recognizing the distance between the two voices that exist within him and he is left unable to decide which voice truly belongs to him, which voice he embodies and controls. This final scene of the play, Knox argues, contains a "renewed insistence on the heroic nature of Oedipus; the play ends as it began, with the greatness of the hero. But it is a different kind of greatness. It is now based on knowledge, not, as before, on ignorance, and this new knowledge is, like that of Socrates, a recognition of man's ignorance" (Knox 1968, p. 97).

Perhaps Oedipus will discover the answers he seeks at Colonus.

Conflicts of Interest: The author declares no conflict of interest.

References

Antze, Paul. 2003. Illness as Irony in Psychoanalysis. In *Illness and Irony: On the Ambiguity of Suffering in Culture.* Edited by Michael Lambek and Paul Antze. New York: Berghahn Books, pp. 102–21.

Aristotle. 1997. *Poetics.* Translated by Samuel H. Butcher. New York: Hill and Wang.

Blanchot, Maurice. 1997. *Friendship.* Translated by Elizabeth Rottenberg. Stanford: Stanford University Press.

Breuer, Josef, and Sigmund Freud. 1961. *Studies in Hysteria.* Translated by Abraham A. Brill. Boston: Beacon Press.

Burke, Kenneth. 1941. Four Master Tropes. *The Kenyon Review* 3: 421–38.

Caruth, Cathy. 1996. *Unclaimed Experience: Trauma, Narrative, and History*. Baltimore and London: Johns Hopkins University Press.

Chase, Cynthia. 1979. Oedipal Textuality: Reading Freud's Reading of Oedipus. *Diacritics* 9: 53–68. [CrossRef]

Freud, Sigmund. 1939. *Moses and Monotheism*. Translated by Katherine Jones. New York: Vintage Books.

Freud, Sigmund. 1940. *The Interpretation of Dreams*. Translated by Abraham A. Brill. New York: Carlton House.

Freud, Sigmund. 1961. *Beyond the Pleasure Principle*. Translated by James Strachey. New York and London: W.W. Norton and Company.

Gould, Thomas. 1970. *Translation with Commentary of Oedipus the King*. Englewood Cliffs: Prentice Hall.

Hölderlin, Friedrich. 1984. In lieblicher Bläue ['In Lovely Blue']. In *Hymns and Fragments*. Translated by Richard Sieburth. Princeton: Princeton University Press, pp. 247–53.

Hölderlin, Friedrich. 1986. Notes on the Oedipus. In *Comparative Criticism, Vol. 5*. Translated by Jeremy Adler. Edited by E. S. Shaffer. Cambridge: Cambridge University Press, pp. 231–37.

Knox, Bernard. 1968. The Last Scene. In *20th-Century Interpretations of Oedipus Rex*. Edited by Michael J. O'Brien. Englewood Cliffs: Prentice-Hall, pp. 90–98.

Knox, Bernard. 1979. *Word and Action: Essays on the Ancient Theater*. Baltimore and London: Johns Hopkins University Press.

Lambek, Michael. 2003. Introduction: Irony and Illness—Recognition and Refusal. *Social Analysis: The International Journal of Social and Cultural Practice* 47: 1–19. [CrossRef]

Pucci, Pietro. 1988. Reading the Riddles of Oedipus Rex. In *Language and the Tragic Hero*. Edited by Pietro Pucci. Atlanta: Scholars Press, pp. 131–54.

Rokem, Freddie. 1996. One Voice and Many Legs: Oedipus and the Riddle of the Sphinx. In *Untying the Knot: On Riddles and Other Enigmatic Modes*. Edited by Galit Hasan-Rokem and David Shulman. Oxford: Oxford University Press, pp. 255–70.

Sophocles. 1984. *Oedipus the King*. Translated by Robert Fagles. New York: Penguin Books.

Vernant, Jean-Pierre. 1978. Ambiguity and Reversal: On the Enigmatic Structure of *Oedipus Rex*. Translated by Page DuBois. *New Literary History* 9: 475–501. [CrossRef]

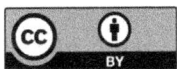

humanities

MDPI

Article

Children and Trauma: Unexpected Resistance and Justice in Film and Drawings

Cheri M. Robinson

Department of Spanish & Portuguese, University of California, Los Angeles, CA 90095-1532, USA;
cherirob7@g.ucla.edu

Received: 22 November 2017; Accepted: 14 February 2018; Published: 26 February 2018

Abstract: This transnational study examines representations of and by children—whether literal wounds, psychological ones, or wounds transmitted through drawings—that manifest their capacity for unexpected resistance and justice. It considers the Mexican-American director Guillermo del Toro's use of hauntings and wounds to explore violence during the 1936–1939 Spanish Civil War in the film *El espinazo del diablo* [*The Devil's Backbone*] (2001) and its intersections on strategic and theoretical levels with the traumatic in archival children's drawings produced during the 1976–1983 Argentine military dictatorship. The drawings illustrate the violence perpetrated against the child artists' families and were produced in exile for the human rights organization COSOFAM. Utilizing diverse theories from film and trauma studies, among others, this article analyzes key scenes in *El espinazo* exhibiting commonalities with representations of traumatic violence in the children's drawings, revealing that, in fiction and in fact, a strategic "showing" of the traumatic wound is designed to remind others of the imperative to intervene in situations of extreme violence, to appeal to/for justice, and to effectively testify from the inside.

Keywords: film; archival drawings; human rights; representations of traumatic violence; children; transnational

---

This transnational study analyzes hauntings and wounds in the Mexican-American director Guillermo del Toro's fictional interpretation of violence during the Spanish Civil War (1936–1939) in the film *El espinazo del diablo* [*The Devil's Backbone*] (2001) and its intersections with representations of traumatic violence during the Argentine military dictatorship (1976–1983) in archival children's drawings.[1] The archival drawings illustrate violence—armed guards, prison bars and cells, captives (almost exclusively women and children)—perpetrated against the child artists' families.[2] Produced in exile in the Netherlands for the human rights organization COSOFAM or the *Comisión de Solidaridad con Familiares de Desaparecidos en Argentina* [Commission of Solidarity with Family Members of those Disappeared in Argentina], the drawings in my view represent the traumatic highlighting of state violence and a cry for justice, which I posit intersects with del Toro's representational strategies. The artistic representations in both instances work through a "showing" of the wound, an appeal to/for

---

[1] IMPORTANT NOTE: Pictures of the archival drawings were obtained with the permission of the *Archivo Nacional de la Memoria* [National Archive of Memory] in Argentina and cannot be reproduced for monetary gain or without authorization. I have not included the drawings within the text due to restrictions regarding their dissemination.

[2] According to the *Catálogo de Fondos Escritos/Audiovisuales/Fotográficos* [Catalogue of Written/ Audiovisual/Photographic Collections] (Alicia Raquel Puchulu de Drangosch Archive 2014), Alicia Raquel Puchulu de Drangosch founded and was president of COSOFAM in the Netherlands during the Argentine military dictatorship. She was forced to flee Argentina to ensure her and her family's safety. I discovered the children's drawings/postcards in her archive, part of a collection donated in 2014 by her daughters to the *Archivo Nacional de la Memoria* in Buenos Aires, thanks to the Ben and Rue Pine travel grant (2015).

justice, and potentially catharsis.[3] At least two films connected to del Toro, *El espinazo del diablo* [*The Devil's Backbone*] (2001) and *El orfanato* [*The Orphanage*] (2007), employ phantoms and children's drawings to "show" hidden violence and unresolved injustices.[4] This study refers to the wounded child phantom Santi and the orphan Jaime's drawing of his murdered body in *El espinazo* and their potential intersections with the archival drawings on strategic and theoretical levels.[5] Otherwise stated, drawings in both instances employ similar strategies and functions to unveil violence and seek justice, demonstrating children's agency in the process.

These representations of and by children—whether literal wounds, psychological ones, or wounds transmitted through drawings—manifest children's capacity for unexpected resistance and justice. In both del Toro's fictional interpretation and the Argentine/Dutch human rights campaign—a campaign in which children were simply instructed, "Hagan dibujos sobre la situación en Argentina" ['Draw about the situation in Argentina'] (Moyano 2016)—children testify of violence.[6] Although the child artists in the Netherlands were asked to create drawings about the situation in Argentina—per my correspondence with E. Moyano, the granddaughter of the founder of COSOFAM and one of the child artists,—they were not told specifically what to draw, just as the child artist in *El espinazo* also chose what he would represent.[7] As such, their representational choices are ones based on free will and, in this article, choice is tied to agency. The child artists, though very young, possessed knowledge of (had witnessed) the violence that forced their families to flee Argentina; the orphans in *El espinazo* also developed a painful awareness of the violence tearing their world apart as they witnessed it and were wounded by it. This traumatic knowledge positions the children in both *El espinazo* and the Netherlands as agents capable of choosing based upon a *full knowledge of the traumatic*.

The archival drawings were imprinted on postcards that were mailed by COSOFAM and others in the Netherlands to the President of the Supreme Court of Justice, D. Adolfo Gabrielli, at the Palace of Justice in the Argentine Federal Capital and possibly to other unknown recipients. According to A. Calvo, an employee at the *Archivo Nacional de la Memoria*, these kinds of postcards were commonly produced to be sent to judges, military personnel, priests, or Argentine authority figures, among others, by parties sympathetic to human rights work and/or overtly against the military dictatorship (Calvo 2016).[8] Calvo remarked that campaigns of this sort were used to pressure authorities from abroad, and it is possible that other sets of postcards were mailed from the Netherlands (Calvo 2016). Moyano was eight or nine years old when the drawings were created and was aware they were to be made into postcards, although she did not know if they were part of fundraising activities for the organization or if they were mailed to other organizations like the United Nations (Moyano 2016). According to Calvo and the information on the postcards, it is clear they were mailed to a judge. Therefore, the archival drawings are categorized as (artistic publicity) "exposing" the dictatorship, which situates them as unique tools demonstrating the violation of human rights through children's personal experiences with state violence. When viewed as tools that expose concealed violence, they then serve the same function as the diegetic drawings in *El espinazo*. It is pertinent to mention that,

---

3   My initial research findings on the comparative study of children's drawings in del Toro's films and those from the archive in Argentina were first presented at the ACLA Annual Meeting at Harvard University in 2016. Since then, I have altered and expanded upon my initial conclusions based on new information.
4   This theme of the traumatic past/phantoms haunting the present is represented in *El orfanato* (2007), directed by J.A. Bayona with del Toro as an executive producer.
5   I recognize that many scholars might disagree with my decision to juxtapose representational strategies and purposes of a fictional interpretation with archival drawings, and I want to emphasize that my intention is to place them in dialogue with each other, not to suggest that the Spanish Civil War and the Argentine military dictatorship were the same. They are distinct historical events, but that does not mean reconstructions of violence pertaining to either period cannot pursue similar strategies or purposes.
6   Translations from Spanish to English are mine; please note that I have attempted to maintain the original meanings instead of translating word for word.
7   Names of personal correspondents have been shortened for privacy.
8   Information was also obtained via email from I. Suarez. "Archivo nacional de la memoria—Cartas postales de COSOFAM." Email message to author, 27 May and 14 September 2016.

although the grounding of human rights on one's humanity is a common assumption, it has failed to hold true in many instances initially discussed by theorists such as Hannah Arendt (Arendt 1958, pp. 291–92) who claimed that the rights of man, with the growing problem of statelessness, were found to be tied to established governments, not to the individual.

The archival drawings, when seen as a response to a reorganizational process in Argentina tied to annihilation as a tool of social engineering (Feierstein 2014), become more than isolated incidents of violence, more than decontextualized images, or simple revelations. They instead take on additional meaning as a *haunting* of the disappeared victim—by revealing concealed violence and calling for an outside recognition of injustice (while abuses were still occurring in Argentina, prior to full-exposure) in much the same way that the murdered child Santi becomes visible through a drawing and his haunting of the orphanage (while violence continues to unfold, prior to the murderer's exposure). The drawings demonstrate the resilience of the "memory" of those disappeared and appropriated, a memory that continues to resist discourses of exclusion, as the past continually revisits (haunts) the present each time the drawings are viewed.

Is a drawing, much like a photograph or the image of Santi's wounded body (in Jaime's drawing and as a phantom), still powerful whether decontextualized or recontextualized? In her essay on "Cuerpos políticos/Body Politics," Taylor (2009) references Fernando Gutiérrez's photograph "Cosas del río" ['River Things'], her friend (viewing the photo) Mario Bronfman's connection to exile, and the photograph's decontextualized images that were nonetheless powerful in their symbolism:

> Photography, the art of de- and re-contextualizing, can isolate and freeze the moment, much in the way that violence ruptures our present from our past and freezes time in a simple before/after ... The violent separation of each object, bracketed off from the rest, also invokes the pain and isolation of exile, the life lived out of place. The photograph unsettles–showing simultaneously too little and too much. (Taylor 2009, p. 22).

The children's drawings, much the same as the photographs and the image of the wounded child, also show too little and too much, but the power of these images remains undeniable. They evoke an emotional response even when standing alone, and emotion draws the viewer in—counteracting a potentially disinterested or distant stance. They serve as a silent witness of the child artists' traumatic pasts and validate pain—potentially with or without a narrative attached to them. However, as with the following analysis of del Toro's film and the situation of the traumatic within a narrative of sense (narrative memory + the restoration of sense), I have chosen to contextualize the drawings separately from the film by providing information obtained from the Archive and personal correspondence.

In lieu of fictional works distorting or distracting from the actual act of bearing witness to violence, filmic fiction can serve a purpose parallel to that of artistic representation, whether utilized as an appeal to/for justice (through the exposure of acts of violence) or as catharsis (a means of "working-through" the traumas of one's past or present). Concerning catharsis, C. Gardner, an employee at South Coast Hospice in Oregon, informed me that art is often used as therapy for children (Gardner 2017). She indicated that their former Light House Program, a support/grief group whose purpose was to assist children who had lost a loved one or experienced a traumatic event that they were unable to adequately describe in words, employed art, collages, crafts, and games (Gardner 2017). In the case of the Light House Program, as with the diegetic drawing, which Jaime creates after witnessing Santi's murder, art may be viewed as a purposeful return to the place of trauma to aid healing or as a "coming to terms" for a grieving or traumatized individual.

Representations of the Traumatic

Carolina Rocha and Georgia Seminet group *El espinazo del diablo* within a category of films that present "the trend depicting the war years and the Franco dictatorship" from the perspective of children and adolescents: "First, preadolescent children are much more frequently cast in filmic narratives constructed on historical memory and trauma" (Rocha and Seminet 2012, p. 4). They describe the film as follows: "Characterized as a transnational film par excellence, *El espinazo* takes place in an orphanage that acts as a 'microcosm for the conflict taking place outside'" (Rocha and Seminet 2012, p. 11). From this standpoint, the traumatic events within the orphanage—tensions between the teachers and young boys (supporters or children of Republicans) & Jacinto, a former orphan who turns against the orphanage for greed, and his thuggish accomplices (potentially the Nationalist band, potentially simple profiteers)—mirror the conflict without, the struggle between the Republicans (loyal to the Second Republic) and the Nationalists (led by General Francisco Franco) (Lázaro-Reboll 2007). This study focuses on the war within and the wounds resulting from the betrayals and murders committed by Jacinto.

The viewer first witnesses the body of the wounded child in the initial sequence. The sequence is a series of five shots, connected by the voice-over of Dr. Casares and a dissolve from the fourth to the fifth shot, exploring the meaning of a phantom:

> DR. CASARES. ¿Qué es un fantasma? Un evento terrible condenado a repetirse una y otra vez. Un instante de dolor, quizás. Algo muerto que parece por momentos vivo aún. Un sentimiento suspendido en el tiempo, como una fotografía borrosa, como un insecto atrapado en ámbar.

> DR. CASARES. What is a phantom? A terrible event condemned to repeat itself time after time. An instant of pain, perhaps. Something dead that at times seems still alive. A sentiment suspended in time, like a blurred photograph, like an insect trapped in amber. (*El espinazo del diablo* [*The Devil's Backbone*] 2001).

The voice-over is repeated at the end of the film with an additional line revealing the Doctor's own connection to phantoms. The film's narration, mostly linear and chronological except for several flashbacks, is united by the repetition of the beginning voice-over, paired with a new set of shots, at the end. The initial establishing sequence begins with a slow movement towards a darkened doorway ["¿Qué es un fantasma? Un evento terrible condenado a repetirse una y otra vez."], then cuts [sound of the cargo doors opening] to the underside of a plane as the cargo doors open and a bomb drops into a rain-filled sky illuminated by various explosions and fires on the ground. The shot ends with the closing of the cargo doors, and the next one starts with the image of a wounded child (later identified as Santi) lying on the ground ["Un instante de dolor, quizás."]. His head has a large gash that is bleeding out onto the ground as another boy (later revealed to be Jaime) touches the wound, bloodying his own fingers and face in the process, and cries ["Algo muerto que parece por momentos vivo aún."]. The fourth shot is of a murky body of water with an initially unknown object that appears to be sinking ["Un sentimiento suspendido en el tiempo,"]. A boy's face is finally visible ["como una fotografía borrosa,"], his body descending deeper into the water, while the camera moves up and outside of the water to show the older boy from the third shot, still crying, as he gazes into the body of water, now visibly a cistern ["como un insecto atrapado en ámbar."]. The fourth shot is connected to the fifth, final shot as the cistern scene dissolves into another murky fluid with unrecognizable objects floating in it. These objects are eventually identified as fetuses with exposed spinal cords or spina bifida, an allusion to the devil's backbone from which the film derives its name.

This initial sequence firmly links *El espinazo* to the imagery of trauma: (1) The darkened doorway or entrance into the traumatic, the unknown, and death; (2) the bomb or harbinger of death (condemned to repeat itself); (3) the moment of trauma or the wound of the child; (4) the place of trauma or the scene of the crime and its concealment; and (5) the open wounds on the bodies of the fetuses. With these images and Dr. Casares's question/response in mind, the viewer delves into del Toro's traumatic world as the images, pieces to a larger puzzle, are explored and slowly fitted together to form a more cogent picture of the moment of trauma.

Scholar and trauma theorist Cathy Caruth describes trauma as an unassimilated event that extends beyond a simple violent act:[9]

> Just as Tancred does not hear the voice of Clorinda until the second wounding, so trauma is not locable in the simple violent or original event in an individual's past, but rather in the way that its very unassimilated nature–the way it was precisely *not known* in the first instance–returns to haunt the survivor later on. (Caruth 1996, p. 4).

The wound and the voice that cries out from it are tied to the belatedness of trauma, its unassimilated nature, and its being *not known* at the moment of wounding; for these reasons, the "missed" trauma may return to haunt those who survive the initial wounding (p. 4). *El espinazo* revisits a past violence through the phantom child's return to (his haunting of) the place of trauma (a concealed murder). The use of wounded phantoms in the film is literally a return to the haunting of trauma in trauma studies. The traumatic is given materiality in the frightful appearance of the wounded phantom child Santi while the abject that produces repulsion is also unexpectedly re-appropriated as both a warning of future violence and a cry for justice for past violence. Through traumatic imagery, Santi and the other orphans are converted into sites of traumatic memory (symbolically) and (literal agents of) justice, one founded in natural law and the supernatural—both of which must serve the victims in the absence of positive laws and guardians to protect them.

Santi, although a phantom seen by a child, appears as more than an inner fantasy; he also bears the marks of an outer violence that takes on physicality in his labored breathing and profusely bleeding head wound. Santi's pain circulates through an aching of the senses and a presentation of grotesque violence—a brutality that causes the spectator to cringe. The use of affect is striking and necessary, a shock linked to sense and justice. This justice will be brought to Santi through the intercession of the main protagonist, Carlos, who will witness and know the site of the unknown trauma—unassimilated but not unwitnessed by Jaime, an older boy at the orphanage present at the time of Santi's murder, who initially remains silent yet draws the murdered boy with a head gash in his sketchbook. Returning to the "originary meaning of trauma" as corporeal (Caruth 1996, p. 3), the haunting of the traumatic becomes more than a wounded mind; it is also externalized in a boy and his wounded, slain body or other mutilated and murdered bodies—all peopling the landscape of Civil War Spain. To "know" the trauma of the phantom child, of the children and teachers killed in the orphanage, Carlos and the orphans must recognize the significance of the open wound and return to the site of violence to bear witness and bring justice. This process of recognition and return works to reestablish equilibrium and sense and to reincorporate traumatic memory back into narrative memory (Van der Kolk and van der Hart 1995, pp. 158–82) by *knowing* the belatedness inherent in the original moment of trauma.

The wound acts as a testimony of unresolved violence in the manners in which it is presented to Carlos and the viewer. Scholar Adriana Bergero argues that the abject circulates, attempting to diminish the distance between it and the living: "En la escena gótica-film de horror y para el estupor de los vivos, el monstruo abyecto se constituye como un *otro* inconveniente que circula ansioso por acercar distancias con los vivos" ['In the gothic scene/horror film and to the amazement of the living, the abject monster constitutes itself as an inconvenient *other* that circulates, anxious to move closer to the living'] (Bergero 2010, p. 443). Throughout the film, the attempt to establish contact and diminish distance occurs first on Santi's part and finally on the part of Carlos. There is a gradual movement from repulsion to solidarity: from sight to touch and from aversion to empathy and understanding.

Santi first appears to Carlos in the daylight. He is viewed from a distance, and the contact is based on *sight* alone. The viewer, but not Carlos, is privy to a shot of Santi's face through a dirty window.

---

[9]   Caruth appropriates the symbols of the wound and the voice from Freud's analysis of a story, recounted by Tasso in the epic *Gerusalemme Liberata* [*Jerusalem Delivered*] (1581), about the knight Tancred who accidentally wounds his beloved Clorinda (Caruth 1996, p. 2).

Insects are flying around him, and he appears destitute. Carlos is still unaware that the boy he saw is a phantom, but the viewer is now cognizant of the figure's abnormal appearance. Santi's second contact with Carlos is through Carlos's physical connection with his former sleeping area (bed number 12); he responds with a murmur when his name is spoken aloud (*sound*).[10] Carlos sees Santi's shadow again, but this time the shadow reaches out to him as Carlos asks him who he is. Santi proceeds to knock over the water pitcher at the end of the bed, and as the water spills onto the floor (perhaps an allusion to the cistern) his retreating footprints are visible on the wet floor. Santi's attempt to establish contact is again interrupted by the approach of the other orphans.

In the kitchen scene where Carlos and Jaime are filling their water pitchers, Santi approaches Carlos again with a whisper of his name (*sound*). As he descends the stairs into the cistern room, a shadow runs by, and there is a brief close-up shot of Santi's wounded and decaying face. Santi appears behind Carlos; as he touches Carlos's arm, he screams and disappears (*touch* and *sound*). Santi has crossed the barrier; he has transitioned from *sight* to *sound* to *touch*. He also leaves a trace of the blood from his wound in the air, blood that is touched and rubbed between Carlos's fingers, testing its materiality. A voice-off of Santi is heard, "Muchos van a morir" ['Many are going to die']. He sounds as if he were struggling for breath, but his words are still perceived as a threat, not yet a warning. When Carlos again flees, Santi attempts to follow him. He ascends the stairs while Carlos is struggling to squeeze outside of the locked door. Santi may have eliminated the physical distance separating him from Carlos in the cistern room, but he is still far from effectively communicating. His abject appearance repulses instead of inspiring pity. The absence of empathy and sense is firmly in place.

Sociologist Gabriel Gatti speaks of the forced disappearances of people as catastrophes that occurred in the terrain of sense and especially affected identity and language (Gatti 2011, p. 85). While the archival drawings certainly fit within the category of "catastrophe" as they display violence enacted against families that resulted in the forced disappearances of loved ones (inexpressible acts affecting familial ties), Santi's trauma is not necessarily in the traditional arena of the disappeared, in the Southern Cone sense—although he is believed missing or considered a runaway before his murder is discovered. However, it does share some common characteristics when viewed through the lens of the more universal description of a *desaparecido* ['a forcibly disappeared person'] (Gatti 2011, p. 228). Essentially, *el desaparecido modélico* [the prototypical *desaparecido*] (again, in the Southern Cone sense) has evolved into *el desaparecido transnacional* ['the transnational *desaparecido*'] which in turn has been re-appropriated in *el desaparecido local* ['the local *desaparecido*'] (p. 221). The archival drawings fall within the concept of *el desaparecido modélico*; whereas, in Santi's case, the re-appropriation of *el desaparecido local* occurs in the figure of the wounded orphan—a defenseless child made more vulnerable by his exposure to the violence of civil war and those like Jacinto who take advantage of the dismantling of protective structures. Where the archival drawings and filmic representations of the traumatic both meet (in a contemporary context) is in the concept of *el desaparecido transnacional*, elaborated in international human rights legislation in organizations like the United Nations, to which COSOFAM was potentially appealing, and other human rights groups whose description of the concept later expands to include marginalized/socially invisible persons like the boys in the orphanage.[11]

Gatti's elaboration on the evolution of the term *desaparecido* also includes a restitution of sense to an act, *desaparición forzada* ['forced disappearance'], that dismantles the links of identity, family, community, and language (p. 85). The act represents the absence of sense. I propose that del Toro utilizes representational strategies (hauntings and open wounds on the bodies of orphans) and the language of affect—or more specifically the emotions of horror, fear, and pain, along with the pursuit of justice—to restore sense to the broken body of a child. By considering the language of affect as a restoration of sense in the film, I believe Gatti's proposition that one's reaction to absence, emptiness,

---

10 Carlos pronounces the name "Santi," carved on the wall by the bed.
11 One example is the International Convention for the Protection of All Persons from Enforced Disappearance (December 2006).

and a lack of sense is "to fill it with sense" (*llenarlo de sentido*) provides an intriguing rationale for the use of horror or the gothic to revisit the traumatic past (p. 88).

The term *desaparecido/a* has evolved into a referent for those terrible, exceptional situations that pose problems of referentiality: "En fin, diría que hoy el desaparecido cataliza las hablas de *la lengua de lo ausente del sentido*" ['In short, I would say that today the desaparecido, or figure of the forcibly disappeared person, catalyzes the speech of *the language of the absence of sense*'] (emphasis Gatti's) (Gatti 2011, p. 229). Gatti describes the term's broad applicability as if it were a substitute for that which has no name or place, "Y en la medida que el desaparecido se eleva a ese lugar, el de referencia, metáfora, concepto, el lenguaje que fue útil para hablarlo se convierte también en el lenguaje de esas *cosas sin nombre ni lugar*" ['And to the extent that the desaparecido is raised to that place, that of reference, metaphor, concept, the language that was useful to speak of it is also converted into the language of those *things without name or place*'] (emphasis Gatti's, p. 229). In *El espinazo*'s exhibition of the child's wounded body, the intolerable image fills in as a metaphor or visual language to reveal an environment defined by a void of sense and empathy that creates a fertile ground for the propagation of violence and, in the displaying of the intolerable image, for the filling of this vacuum with an overabundance of sense and emotion. In the orphanage, the ties linking the children to their families and communities have been broken by war and death; they are fragments of a larger whole that has been dismantled by the violence of civil war. In such an environment, full of pain, the phantom child returns to remind Carlos that his wounds are crying out. Santi's body serves as a testimony to the materiality of the trauma he suffered, and his wounds shock the desensitized viewer into feeling.

The child's battered body is visually intolerable in its all "too real" depiction of reality. I propose that the graphic nature of the wounded body falls under Jacques Ranciere's analysis of the "shift from the intolerable in the image to the intolerability of the image" (Ranciere 2009, pp. 83–84). Although the wounded orphans and Santi's abject appearance provoke the aversion of the viewer's gaze, just as they initially evoke Carlos's fear and desire to flee, the purpose of displaying such brutality is precisely to remove the traumatic event from its state of isolation and to restore sense to the absence of sense. The intolerable image is contextualized; it serves a purpose. The reincorporation of traumatic histories and the restoration of sense occur in the situating of the intolerable image within the sequence of events that made it intolerable, not in its situation as an isolated event that would possibly lead to its intolerability. The intolerability of the image is displaced by "the construction of the victim as an element in a certain distribution of the visible. An image never stands alone" (Ranciere 2009, p. 99). The abject appearance of Santi's wounded body is intolerable, as are the images of violence in the archival drawings created by children, but the open wound or mark of violence serves the purpose of drawing one's attention to an *unknown* trauma.

In the aftermath of the tragic explosion caused by Jacinto, Jaime finally speaks of Santi's murder. There is a flashback to the cistern room as Jaime verbally revisits the scene of the crime: (1) Jaime comes out of hiding—after Jacinto pushes Santi into a pillar and wounds his head—and bends over Santi to touch his bleeding forehead, and (2) Jaime comes out of hiding again—after Jacinto weighs down Santi's body and throws it into the water—to crouch in front of the cistern and cry. The bomb falls out of the sky as Jaime leaves the murder scene and walks into the courtyard. Carlos and the viewer—through the testimony of the witness Jaime (visual and verbal) and the approach of the wounded phantom—have now returned to the scene of the crime and witnessed its occurrence. As such, the history of the trauma is no longer *unknown*. Armed with the knowledge of the traumatic, Carlos can approach Santi without fleeing, without aversion to his repulsive appearance, because he recognizes and hears the crying wound.

Carlos progresses from a reactive stance to a proactive one towards the phantom presence as he recognizes that the lack of justice must be filled with justice, the lack of empathy with emotion, and the absence of assistance with action, yet he does not act alone. Jaime also realizes that his fear must be replaced with courage, since no one will fight for him and the other orphans; they must fight for themselves. Jacinto, lured into the cistern room, initially laughs at the sight of little boys armed with skinny sticks, but his laughter is shortly converted to pain as Jaime takes the first shot, stabbing him underneath the arm. As the boys use superior numbers to their advantage, they continually pierce Jacinto's body with their sticks until he is close enough to be shoved into the cistern. Santi is now free to claim his justice, a death for a death. The children, standing in front of the water with their bloodied sticks, have revisited the place of trauma and assisted the phantom. Not only has Santi's traumatic history been resituated within the broader narrative of the orphans' stories, but justice has been restored to an environment devoid of it.

There is no happy ending or airtight resolution in the film, but there are necessary restitutions. There is no guarantee that the orphans make it to town or find the nurture and assistance they so desperately require, but they have survived by moving from the sidelines of the battle to its forefront in their decision to assist Santi. Although it may seem shocking to call Jacinto's death justice instead of murder, it is also an act that occurs in an environment of ultimate impunity, one in which there is no formal legal system and no surviving guardians to whom the orphans can appeal. Regardless of their response to the cry of the phantom child, they still would have had to resort to a defensive violence to survive Jacinto's brutality. In the film, the lines between justice and vengeance blur due to the exceptional circumstances existing in the orphanage; the orphans are given no other recourse than to meet violence with violence or be killed.

In addition to my proposition that Jaime's drawing in *El espinazo* be considered for its potential cathartic properties and its signaling of a hidden crime, I suggested that the archival children's drawings be viewed as artistic publicity for human rights. This would also identify the drawings as the representation of a reprehensible crime (forced disappearance) in addition to a call for intervention, both characteristics shared with the diegetic drawing and wounded phantom. It is possible that the concept of art as catharsis may also be relevant to the archival drawings, since the children who participated in the project were Puchulu de Drangosch's grandchildren (ranging in age from five to nine years old), all of whom had experienced the violence of forced disappearance and appropriation firsthand (Moyano 2016).[12] However, because Moyano indicated that the children were asked to draw pictures about the situation in Argentina, the work of catharsis, if applicable, and human rights are performed simultaneously. Whatever their function or purpose, the archival drawings also demand an accounting in their display of intolerable images reinforced by a naming of the individuals missing.

Of the eight, six of the illustrated postcards were connected to demands to know the whereabouts of "kidnapped" (forcibly disappeared or missing) children and two were tied to "kidnapped" pregnant women. The text on the backs of all eight begins with the phrase, "Con todo respeto, pero con todo dolor, queremos saber" ['With all due respect, but with much sorrow, we want to know'], which is then followed by one of two questions. For the postcards concerning "kidnapped" children, the demand is typed in all capital letters and reads, "DONDE ESTAN LOS NINOS SECUESTRADOS POR EL GOBIERNO ARGENTINO" ['Where are the children kidnapped by the Argentine government']. For those postcards referring to "kidnapped" pregnant women, the demand reads, "DONDE ESTAN LAS MUJERES EMBARAZADAS SECUESTRADAS POR EL GOBIERNO ARGENTINO" ['Where are the pregnant women kidnapped by the Argentine government']. The demand is then reiterated in Dutch and followed by a list of three names on each postcard with either the ages of the children/adolescents or the number of months the women were pregnant. In both cases, the emphasis is on the children/adolescents and fetuses, a focus evident in the children's drawings.[13]

In her analysis of Felman and Laub's seminal work on the Holocaust (Felman and Laub 1992), Kelly Oliver describes the necessity of bearing witness from the inside (declared impossible when the addressable other is abolished, as occurred in concentration camps) to the re-establishment of

---

12   The child artists were Moyano, her sisters, and cousin.
13   Several supporting entities are also listed: CO. SO. FAM. (COSOFAM), A.F.U.D.E., *Nederlandse Kinderraad* [Netherlands Council for Children], *Komitee Twee* [Committee Two], *Kerk en Vrede* [Church and Peace], I.F.O.R., *Stichting Oecumenische Hulp* [Foundation for Ecumenical Assistance], *Kerken en Vluchtelingen* [Churches and Refugees], and N.C.O., respectively.

subjectivity (Oliver 2001). In turn, witnessing and subjectivity are connected to justice and require another person (who will respond and be responsible) to claim it:

> Yet in order to reestablish subjectivity and in order to demand justice, it is necessary to bear witness to the inarticulate experience of the inside. . . . It is the tension between finite understanding linked to historical facts and historically determined subject positions, and the infinite encounter linked to psychoanalysis and the infinite responsibility of subjectivity that produces a sense of agency. Such an encounter necessarily takes us beyond recognition and brings with it ethical obligation. (Oliver 2001, p. 90).

The children's drawings have the power of expressing the inexpressible (*to bear witness to the inarticulate experience of the inside*)—connected to subjectivity (requires the possibility of a witness for Oliver), response-ability, ethical obligations, and justice. For Oliver, "Response-ability is never solitary" (p. 91) (unlike the traumatic narrative addressed to no one). The drawings, when viewed as symbolic expressions of "the inside," request and require an audience who will be ethically responsible.

Building on Dori Laub's idea of an "inner witness" or addressable other, Oliver postulates:

> To conceive of oneself as a subject is to have the ability to address oneself to another, real or imaginary, actual or potential. Subjectivity is the result of, and depends on, the process of witnessing—address-ability and response-ability. Oppression, domination, enslavement, and torture work to undermine and destroy the ability to respond and there-by undermine and destroy subjectivity. (Oliver 2001, p. 17).

In this context, the drawings can function as a means for children to address themselves to others and for human rights organizations through children to work against the forces of violence—the annihilation of social relations and of existence itself. Feierstein (2014) speaks of disappearance as more than murder in that it is an obliteration of one's existence. As a means of resisting the obliteration of the Other and as a reclamation of existence, the drawings attest to a violence that "disappeared" people. They are a tool employed to counteract the process of annihilation and re-establish subjectivity through a confirmation of address-ability and response-ability by "bear[ing] witness to the inarticulate experience of the inside" (Oliver 2001, p. 90).

If civilizing discourses are really discourses of exclusion, a making invisible of those in plain sight, then the dictatorship took this a step further by attempting to render invisible non-conforming citizens, conveniently labeled subversives (rendering them non-citizens and thus without the Rights guaranteed citizens by their government), through their "disappearance" (an initial Othering of people that later develops in certain places into forcibly disappearing the Othered). Arendt analyzed the contradiction inherent in barbarous acts that arise and are sustained by the ubiquitous spread of civilization and argued that "only with a completely organized humanity could the loss of home and political status become identical with expulsion from humanity altogether" (Arendt 1958, p. 297). The reorganizing discourse (*el proceso de reorganización nacional* or the National Reorganization Process) of the dictatorship, bolstered by the underlying civilizing discourse of the Nation, created categorizations or artificial boundaries as a means of isolating and Othering, a process that facilitated genocide as social practice.

Feierstein propagates a model that views "genocide not only as a latent potential of modernity but as [what he terms] a specific technology of power." For Feierstein, "A technology of power is a form of social engineering that creates, destroys, or reorganizes relationships within a given society." He postulates, "It influences the ways in which different social groups construct their identity, the identity of others, and the otherness of the Other, thus shaping the way that groups can relate to themselves and to one another" (Feierstein 2014, p. 1). By closely tying together genocide and social reorganization, genocide (in addition to its legal definition) emerges as a social practice in historical and sociological discourses (Feierstein 2014, p. 14). To push for the adoption of the Genocide Convention, Raphael Lemkin, who coined the word genocide, allowed for the exclusion of political groups, an exclusion that has now problematized the prosecuting of genocide in cases where persecution is tied to political groups or "doing" instead of existential reasons or "being" (Feierstein 2014, p. 32).

The drawings have the potential to fight against the trivialization and normalization of violence by reminding those in positions of power that even children had witnessed Argentine state-sponsored violence, and they had not forgotten it. During the military dictatorship, many of these facts were known and not known (such as the existence of camps) by an Argentine populace paralyzed by fear, and so it was important to continually point to crimes the State was still in the process of concealing.[14] Pilar Calveiro states, "Los militares habían hecho un gran esfuerzo por ocultar o hacer desaparecer los restos de sus víctimas. No sólo habían desaparecido a las personas sino que después desaparecieron a los desaparecidos" ['The military had made a great effort to hide or make the remains of their victims disappear. Not only had they made people disappear but, afterwards, they disappeared the forcibly disappeared'] (Calveiro 1998, p. 163). Drawings, in this case, testify to a violence that sought to annihilate by further disappearing already disappeared lives and bodies. They are a powerful reminder that the children/adolescents and women forcibly disappeared in Argentina might be out of *sight*, but they are certainly not out of *mind/memory*. Their names are known, and their traumatic pasts demand restitution.

Concluding Thoughts on Fiction and the Archive

As mentioned earlier, Jaime's drawing assists Carlos in uncovering Santi's violent death. Santi's body had been pushed into a cistern by Jacinto, effectively hiding or disappearing the murdered boy in the murky water. The drawing thus serves a cathartic purpose by creating a way for Jaime to revisit the site of Santi's death, of which he had not yet spoken, while also pointing to the murder victim. The drawing is Jaime's initial voiceless testimony (from or of the inside), seen in secret by Carlos (who witnesses from the outside). As is evident in *El espinazo* and the archival drawings, children draw what they see. *The drawings visually speak for the victims in that they unveil the unseen and unresolved traumas of the past.* As postulated, this uncovering of the past allows for restitution to occur as the isolated trauma is again situated within a chain of events and narrative:

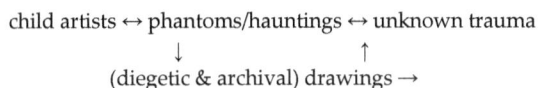

$$\text{child artists} \leftrightarrow \text{phantoms/hauntings} \leftrightarrow \text{unknown trauma}$$
$$\downarrow \qquad\qquad\qquad \uparrow$$
$$\text{(diegetic \& archival) drawings} \rightarrow$$

The idea of haunting as a means of revealing past violence with the clear intent of pursuing justice is particularly evident in *El espinazo*, where Jaime's drawing becomes a tool for natural law that works in tandem with the supernatural (in the absence of positive laws). As the orphans answer the phantom's cry for justice, their bodies, repositories marked by violence, carry traumatic memory forward to a final reckoning in which the traumatized child's body is also the weapon or force that claims justice. With the archival children's drawings, the use of visual recreations of unresolved past violence is also utilized for the pursuit of a just recognition of wrongs committed, although within the framework of positive law and human rights work in exile. The archival drawings, as a call for response-ability and address-ability, pursue justice through COSOFAM's propagation of interventionist strategies (using children's drawings to expose violence and request intervention) and demand for accountability on the part of the Argentine State for the "missing" bodies connected to the names listed on the postcards. I have not currently located a document at the Archive stating that any action was taken on the part of the judge in question, but it is possible that a record exists. This would be an intriguing line of inquiry for future studies.

In conclusion, in both fiction and the archive, children actively unveil past violence and demand an accounting. Their drawings "show" the crime. Children become the bearers and transmitters of traumatic memory through hauntings, wounds, and/or drawings. This does not mean that children

---

[14] See also, Marguerite Feitlowitz. 2011. *A Lexicon of Terror: Argentina and the Legacies of Torture, Revised and Updated with a new Epilogue.* Oxford: Oxford University Press.

as the portents of justice must also mete out justice, but in del Toro's film, they do. The weakest and most oppressed victims—orphan children trapped in a state of exception and affected by extreme violence—become agents of restitution and justice, just as Argentine children in exile in the Netherlands actively participated in the fight against state repression by bearing witness of the inside—both acts serving as reminders that "response-ability is never solitary" (Oliver 2001, p. 91).

Acknowledgments: I acknowledge funding I received to do research in Argentina, where I discovered the archival drawings, in footnote 2. I received the Ben and Rue Pine travel grant (summer of 2015).

Conflicts of Interest: The author declares no conflict of interest.

References

Alicia Raquel Puchulu de Drangosch Archive. Donated 2014. *Comisión de Solidaridad con Familiares de Desaparecidos en Argentina* (COSOFAM). Eight Postcards Imprinted with Children's Drawings. No date. Listed in the "Catálogo de Fondos Escritos/Audiovisuales/Fotográficos". Buenos Aires: Archivo Nacional de la Memoria, Accessed on 8 September 2015.

Arendt, Hannah. 1958. *The Origins of Totalitarianism.* Cleveland and New York: Meridian Books, The World Publishing Company.

Bergero, Adriana. 2010. Espectros, escalofríos y discursividad *herida* en *El espinazo del diablo*: El gótico como cuerpo-geografía cognitiva-emocional de quiebre. *No todos los espectros permanecen abandonados. Project Muse* 125: 433–56.

Calveiro, Pilar. 1998. *Poder y Desaparición: Los Campos de Concentración en Argentina.* Buenos Aires: Ediciones Colihue.

Calvo, A. 2016. Archivo Nacional de la Memoria. Email message to author, 7 January.

Caruth, Cathy. 1996. *Unclaimed Experience: Trauma, Narrative, and History.* Baltimore: The Johns Hopkins University Press.

El espinazo del diablo [*The Devil's Backbone*]. 2001. Directed by Toro Guillermo del. Production Companies: El Deseo S.A., Tequila Gang, and Anhelo Producciones. DVD.

Feierstein, Daniel. 2014. *Genocide as Social Practice: Reorganizing Society under the Nazis and Argentina's Military Juntas.* Translated by Douglas Andrew Town. New Brunswick, and London: Rutgers University Press.

Felman, Shoshana, and Dori Laub. 1992. *Testimony: Crises of Witnessing in Literature, Psychoanalysis, and History.* New York and London: Routledge.

Gardner, C. 2017. Light House Program at South Coast Hospice. Email message to author, 28 February.

Gatti, Gabriel. 2011. *Identidades Desaparecidas: Peleas por el Sentido en los Mundos de la Desaparición Forzada.* Buenos Aires: Prometeo Libros.

Lázaro-Reboll, Antonio. 2007. The Transnational Reception of *El espinazo del diablo* (Guillermo del Toro 2001). *Hispanic Research Journal* 8: 39–51. [CrossRef]

Moyano, E. 2016. Suarez del Archivo nacional de la memoria. Email message to author, 16 October.

Oliver, Kelly. 2001. *Witnessing: Beyond Recognition.* Minneapolis and London: University of Minnesota Press.

Ranciere, Jacques. 2009. *The Emancipated Spectator.* Translated by Gregory Elliott. London and New York: Verso.

Rocha, Carolina, and Georgia Seminet. 2012. Introduction. In *Representing History, Class, and Gender in Spain and Latin America: Children and Adolescents in Film.* Edited by Rocha, Carolina and Georgia Seminet. New York: Palgrave Macmillan, pp. 1–29.

Taylor, Diana. 2009. Cuerpos políticos/Body Politics. In *Body Politics: Políticas del Cuerpo en la Fotografía Latinoamericana.* Edited by Brodsky, Marcelo and Julio Pantoja. Buenos Aires: La marca editora, pp. 20–31.

Van der Kolk, Bessel A., and Onno van der Hart. 1995. The Intrusive Past: The Flexibility of Memory and the Engraving of Trauma. In *Trauma: Explorations in Memory.* Edited by Caruth, Cathy. Baltimore and London: The John Hopkins University Press, pp. 158–82.

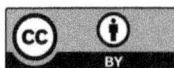

humanities

MDPI

Article

Let Seizing Truths Lie: Witnessing "Factions" in Lauren Slater's *Lying*

Eden Wales Freedman

Department of Communication, Literature and Arts, Mount Mercy University, Cedar Rapids, IA 52402, USA; ewalesfreedman@mtmercy.edu

Received: 11 September 2017; Accepted: 24 October 2017; Published: 31 October 2017

Abstract: In her memoir, *Lying* (2000), Lauren Slater fabricates most of her life narrative. Her text frustrates those who resent the combined fact and fiction—or "faction"—that she spins. This readerly response is understandable. Nevertheless, this article maintains that Slater lies in her memoir not to mislead readers but to witness traumas she struggles to access and articulate. Trauma and autobiographical theorists document the necessity of writing through—or "witnessing"—trauma to overcome it. When, however, a narrator is inhibited by what psychiatrists call "psychic constriction" (memory loss due to an inability to reconcile oneself with a painful past), she can become powerless to take the steps necessary to recover, as she cannot convey fully what she has suffered. Such is the case for Slater, who lies to witness ineffable traumas alongside her very inability to witness them. *Lying* also opens an important question about the reader's role in traumatic witnessing: how does one respond to the traumatic testimony of an unreliable narrator? In answer, inasmuch as one may resist Slater's memoir, one also has the ability to enter into and engage in her experience. In presenting this opportunity, *Lying* offers the writer-narrator and reader-respondent alike, a way to witness trauma together.

Keywords: trauma; memoir; witnessing; *Lying*; reader response

---

In their work with trauma victims, Shoshana Felman and Dori Laub document the necessity of writing through—or "witnessing"—trauma to overcome it. To endure and prevail, they attest, the wounded subject must face her "buried truths" and "piece together" and voice a "fully-realized narrative" (Farrell 1998, p. 1). "The survivor", Laub maintains, must write her story "to survive" (Felman and Laub 1992, p. 63). Autobiographical critic Suzette Henke explains that writing to witness serves as a form of "scriptotherapy," a process that empowers survivors to "write out and through" the traumatic events in their lives (Henke 2001, p. 142). Life-writing, Henke explains, allows the traumatized subject to recall and reframe a once-splintered identity. Through witnessing, a writer serves as both an analyst and analysand of her psychic history; she can then reemerge in written form, as a newly empowered "I" (ibid, p. 142). If a survivor does not write her history, autobiographical theorist and memoirist Janet Ellerby maintains, traumatic aftermath intensifies (Ellerby 2001, p. 25). One may repress a traumatic memory for a period of time, but, until witnessed, the experience continues to haunt.[1]

---

[1]   Recent research on trauma and postcolonial studies (e.g., by Michael Rothberg (Rothberg 2009) and Stef Craps (Craps 2013) has criticized psychoanalytic trauma theory for eliding the traumatic experiences of non-Western or minority groups, by assuming as "universal" a Eurocentric, mono-cultural, logocentric bias, which defines "trauma" as individual and psychoanalytic (versus communal and cultural) and "recovery" as secured exclusively through scriptotherapy (versus other modes, such as dancing, painting, meditation, and/or silence). While I appreciate this critique, this article nevertheless utilizes a psychoanalytic lens to analyze *Lying*, since Slater, a psychoanalyst and a writer, presents her trauma as a unique (or an individual) psychic shattering that calls to be processed through scriptotherapy, versus a larger, cultural catastrophe that could be witnessed in other ways. Given how Slater herself frames her narrative, this article does not debate the merits

In the memoir, *Lying*, author-narrator, Lauren Slater, employs scriptotherapy to witness inaccessible, unknown traumas through the overlapping metaphors of compulsive lying and epileptic seizing. More than the history she struggles to remember and convey, however, Slater's narrative opens certain aporias: what is the reader's role in witnessing? How does one respond to traumatic testimony, particularly when its narrator, like Slater's "Lauren,"[2] admits to being a "slippery sort?" (Slater 2000, p. 160). In answer, inasmuch as a reader may resist *Lying* (a natural response to the tale of a self-described liar and madwoman), one also possesses the opportunity to see through her eyes and read in her voice, and, in doing so, to access and work through her life experiences. That is to say, if a reader can engage in what it feels like to be the writer-narrator, while still sustaining a separate position and individual perspective as a reader-respondent, one can join the writer-narrator in witnessing.

Witnessing, I argue, is not one-sided but interpersonal: The writer-narrator (whom I term the *primary witness*) testifies in relation to the reader-listener (or *secondary witness*) who receives the narrative and attests to its veracity. I call the interchange between writer and reader, *dual-witnessing*, and the failure to engage trauma, *anti-witnessing*.[3] Trauma theorists concur. "It takes two to witness the unconscious," Felman asserts (Felman and Laub 1992, p. 24). Laub corroborates that witnessing requires the "intimate and total presence of an *other*" (ibid, p. 70). In fact, a relational mode is denoted in the definition of the word, "witness." The *Oxford English Dictionary* defines a "witness" as both the speaker who bears witness "from personal observation" (OED 2017c, sense 6a) (the primary witness) and the "spectator or auditor", who bears witness to the speaker's trauma (ibid, sense 6a) (the secondary witness). Accordingly, if Slater is to surmount her trauma, she must do more than write to witness. Readers must witness *Lying*'s contents in return. To clarify, to witness trauma secondarily does not mean that one becomes a survivor oneself. Wendy Hui Kyong Chun explains that the reader engages the writer's "victories, defeats, and silences" and "know[s] them from within" (Chun 2002, p. 162). At the same time, the secondary witness recognizes that she is not the primary witness: she has not suffered precisely what the primary witness has. Dual-witnessing is only possible when a secondary witness engages another's testimony without co-opting it.

For the survivor, the impulse to witness is simultaneously inhibited by what psychiatrist Judith Herman calls "psychic constriction," a state of indeterminate memory loss due to an inability to come to terms with the magnitude of a traumatic event (Herman 1997, p. 42). The constricted narrator, Herman explains, can find herself powerless to take the very steps necessary to recover, since she cannot convey fully what she has suffered (ibid, p. 7). Laub explains that, for traumatized subjects, "there are never enough words or the right words ... to articulate the story that cannot be fully captured" (Felman and Laub 1992, p. 63). However much a narrator may wish to witness, words elude her. The harder she tries, the more difficult witnessing becomes. In attempting to write through trauma, a primary witness may discover that she cannot tell her story; she may not even know what it is.

---

of psychoanalytic trauma theory, or the necessity of scriptotherapy, but explores instead (1) what happens to those, such as Slater, who resonate with writing as a form of psychic healing, but struggle to write through their individual traumas and (2) how readers can respond to such imparted testimony.

2   I refer to the author of *Lying* as "Slater" and call her narrator "Lauren." These figures overlap (both are "Lauren Slater"), and it is not always clear how and when the two diverge and converge. Nevertheless, I wish to distinguish the writer's narrator, "Lauren," from the writer, "Slater," as "Lauren" is a character Slater creates to help her write through an otherwise un-witnessable past, and Slater exists outside of her memoir as the arranger of both "Lauren" and the traumas to which *Lying* testifies.

3   The word "witness" exists as both a noun (the witness) and a verb (to witness). Similarly, the terminology I use to describe dual-witnessing includes both noun and verb forms: one can function as a "primary witness" (n) or secondary witness" (n). One can also "witness primarily" or write through one's traumatic experience (v) and "witness secondarily" or receive another's traumatic testimony (v). An anti-witness (n) refers to a reader-respondent who refuses to engage another's trauma. "To anti-witness" (v) is to disengage from the writer-narrator's traumatic narrative. Autobiographical critics substantiate the dual nature of witnessing. Nancy K. Miller and Jason Tougaw emphasize that witnessing encompasses both the experience of those primary witnesses "who have suffered directly" and those secondary witnesses who "suffer with them, through them, or for them, if only by reading trauma" (Miller and Tougaw 2002, p. 2).

Such is the case for Slater who admits that the "truth" of her history is emblematic, her nonfiction creative. In *Lying*, Slater fuses fact and fiction together into what I call "faction" (an amalgamation of truth and falsehood), because she does not trust her memory. Her inner narrator is unreliable. Slater wants to witness her story, but she cannot extract the truth from the haze of her imaginings. When attempting to recall her history, she confesses: "I had always believed there could be two truths, truth A and truth B". In her experience, however, "A and B were placed in a parallel position, ... so I couldn't decide" what was real and what was not (Slater 2000, p. 94). Slater senses *something* traumatic happened to her, but she cannot work through precisely what that *something* is. She cannot separate A from B to witness either (or something else entirely).

Slater's struggle to separate fact from fiction when witnessing trauma is not unique to her; other memoirists have also explored the notion of "truth" in relation to traumatic memory in their work. Writer Dorothy Allison, for example, has struggled to witness the childhood traumas of physical and sexual abuse and the state-sanctioned stigma of being declared "illegitimate" on her birth certificate. When attempting to write through her trauma, Allison found that language failed to convey adequately her experience. She thus crafted multiple versions of her life story, first using fiction (in the 1992 novel, Bastard out of Carolina), then performance art, and, ultimately, a hybrid memoir, *Two or Three Things I Know for Sure* (Allison 1996), which combined the genres of fiction, performance art, photography, and non-fiction to witness trauma. Together, these texts speak to the continued need to witness in order to heal and the use of multiple genres (and varying, divergent forms of "truth") to do so. Similarly, Susan Brison, a philosophy professor at Dartmouth and a survivor of sexual assault, found the "challenge" of witnessing traumatic experience "daunting" (Brison 2003, p. xi). When she first sat down to write about her rape, she recalls, "things ... stopped making sense" (ibid, ix). "I thought it was quite possible that I was brain-damaged", she confesses. "I couldn't explain what had happened to me" (ibid, ix.) Brison worked through her psychic constriction by publishing a memoir that both details and analyzes from a philosophical perspective, her assault and others' reactions to it. Brison was able to explain what happened (even when language failed her), by periodically stepping out of a traumatic space to analyze from a more distanced, academic perspective how the assault and others' responses to it shaped her traumatic aftermath.

The difference between authors such as Allison and Brison, and Slater, is that Allison and Brison know precisely what happened to them to cause the constriction that hinders scriptotherapy. The narrator in *Lying*, conversely, cannot locate the source of her trauma. Lauren feels compelled to write to witness, but she cannot identify precisely what traumas have shattered her, or how and when they originated. Instead, when asked to diagnose her illness, Lauren becomes constricted. When a police officer inquires whether or not she has epilepsy, she "want[s] to answer," but the words get "tangled in [her] throat" (Slater 2000, p. 43). When prompted to speak about the source of her sickness, she shuts down. Psychic constriction continues throughout *Lying*. A behaviorist encourages Lauren to describe her psychological "triggers"; she "s[ays] nothing" (ibid, p. 37). Her pediatrician asks her to explain what happened to her; she "searche[s] for the words" (ibid, p. 21). Even when Lauren senses she has improved, that "something had changed in me," she cannot witness "exactly what it [is]" (ibid, 56).

The use of "something" and "it" to describe Lauren's condition is significant, in that the pronouns are at once constrictive (indicating an inability to define what *it* is) and open and variable (suggesting that Lauren suffers from anything, everything, and nothing at once). As the English translation of Freud's *id* (Latin: "it"), *it* also expresses Lauren's unconscious, her "repressed [some]things" that, if she could "just let" "fly free" would help her "get better" (ibid, p. 81). While the writer, Slater, artfully conveys Lauren's constricted confusion, the narrator, Lauren, remains unable to decode what *id* is. However much she wishes to witness the "repressed [some]things" of her unconscious, they continue to elude her.

A psychically-constricted Lauren clearly *wants* to witness her traumatic history. When encouraged by friends at an Alcoholics Anonymous meeting to tell her tale—"Lauren, the story saves, Lauren" (ibid, p. 203)—she jumps at the opportunity: "This ... was my chance to tell the truth. "They wanted my story, I would tell them my story" (ibid, p. 203). When she finds herself before the assembly, however, she cannot disclose the workings of her psyche. "In order to do it really right," she realizes "I would also have to admit I was not an alcoholic" (ibid, p. 192). (she has joined the group under false pretenses). Lauren longs to tell her listeners (and Slater longs to tell her readers) that "I suffered from a different disease" (ibid, p. 203), but she does not "really see how that could happen" (ibid, p. 192). Note that, even in disclosing her desire, Lauren does not pronounce what that "different disease" is (ibid, p. 203). She merely repeats that she wants to say *something* that remains unspoken. In this scene, Slater may actually come closer to witnessing than Lauren does, as Lauren fails to speak her trauma (a sense of catastrophe she cannot articulate), while Slater successfully writes through hers (the concurrent desire and inability to witness trauma). While speaking and writing may seem like similar forms of witnessing (both forms testify), psychological trauma and autobiographical theorists maintain that witnessing requires narrators to write, not just speak, through traumatic histories.

When trauma is not witnessed, Herman attests, it "surfaces not as a verbal narrative but as a symptom" (Herman 1997, p. 37), a *something* that manifests, in Lauren's case, as feigned and real seizures, compulsive stealing, and, ultimately, lying—that which helps her gloss over the inscrutabilities with which she wrestles. Lauren constructs fiction to witness truths she can neither access nor articulate. Fittingly, she first supplants truth with metaphor in Literature class, when she tells Sarah Kushner that she is dying of cancer (she is not), so that, out of pity, the popular girls will invite to her to their parties (they do) (Slater 2000, p. 66). From that moment forward, Lauren reconstructs her life through lying. Slater does the same, reminding readers that her memoir's "factions" gesture toward deeper truths. "I'm using metaphor", Slater writes, "specifically the metaphor of epilepsy, to tell my tale, a tale I know no other way of telling, a tale of my past, ... of pains and humiliations and illnesses so subtle and nuanced I could never find the literal words" (ibid, p. 192). Her method becomes "a way of telling you what I have to tell you" (ibid, p. 6), a way to witness traumas that cannot but must be written.

To conflate indefinable trauma with epilepsy, a medical condition that affects other people more than figuratively, risks promoting ableism, the social discrimination against—and associated marginalization and oppression of—persons with disabilities. Ableism defines people according to their (dis)abilities and then classifies those identified as "disabled"—in this case, the epileptic—as inferior to those who are non-disabled (Linton 1998, p. 9). The comparison Slater draws between epilepsy and trauma fosters ableism in suggesting (falsely) that the condition of epilepsy is itself traumatic. Actual epileptics, however, may not classify their neurodiversity as traumatic, but simply as a different way of experiencing the world. The metaphor of epilepsy also encourages an ableist treatment of (and a victim-blaming mentality toward) post-traumatic experience, in linking post-traumatic stress disorder (PTSD) to the medical pathology of an individual, placing the burden of recovery on the "sick" individual, rather than on the conditions that created the trauma. Finally, the seriousness of epilepsy is reduced when Slater ties it to some uncontainable "truth"—especially if that truth is inextricably intertwined with both trauma and falsehood.

The metaphors Slater uses to describe her condition are undoubtedly problematic. Even so, Slater writes figuratively (or lies), not to misappropriate others' experiences or to manipulate her readers, "but for things beyond weight, beyond measure" (Slater 2000, p. 88). She exaggerates to witness unspeakable trauma. Lauren's neurologist, Dr. Neu, tells her: "In one sense you lied, but in another sense you didn't, because ... you were only being true to yourself" (ibid, p. 202). Although Lauren bristles at Neu's characterization, Slater makes a similar point herself. She fashions falsehoods, as if "words might make" that elusive "*it* real" (ibid, p. 14). Her lies point to truth. In this sense, epilepsy marks a fitting metaphor, in Slater's words to "convey"—or witness—"her psyche" (ibid, p. 162). Slater offers the etymology of epilepsy as "com[ing] from the Greek word *epilepsia*, which means 'to take, to seize'" (ibid, p. 71). She does not mention that, in addition to "the act of seizing" (OED 2017a, sense I), epilepsy also depicts "the fact of being seized (ibid, sense 1a). The author's disease thus signifies both its meaning (to seize) and its opposite (to be seized). Few illnesses could better describe Slater's psychic "thrash and spasm" (Slater 2000, p. 81) than one whose appellation is a contronym. Even within its own name, epilepsy denotes where Slater situates Lauren: at the crossroads of multiple discourses. The double meaning of the word "epilepsy" also mirrors the double meaning of the word "witness", a noun and a verb that denotes both the one who speaks or writes through trauma (the primary witness) and the one who engages it (the secondary witness) as well as the act of witnessing (speaking or writing through trauma) and the reception of witnessing (when a reader-listener engages another's traumatic narrative). In this way, the metaphor of epilepsy speaks both to Slater's seizing psychic condition and to the duality inherent in the act of witnessing.

Instead of lying to its readers, then, *Lying* successfully witnesses its writer-narrator's psychic truths. Like Lauren, Slater wants to be understood. She thus witnesses not only why she seizes but why she lies and how her lies function in her memoir. She explains: "If I were making the whole thing up ... I would be doing it not to create a character as a novelist does, but, instead, to create a metaphor that conveys the real person I am" (ibid, p. 162). She later adds: "I do not know how to say the pain directly. I never have" (ibid, p. 204). Through "faction," Slater's memoir metaphorically witnesses a seizing consciousness that transcends language.

Lying depicts symbolic truths, but because Slater has acknowledged this reality—that exaggeration and falsehood are the only "truths" she knows—she is able to witness what would otherwise remain un-witnessable. "I am my best approximation of me," she writes. "I am not a fiction, but nor am I a fact" (ibid, p. 164). Lauren may not be a reliable narrator—there is no way to know which of her stories are factual and/or to what degree—but what Slater, as *Lying*'s arranger, does with her stories becomes more important than whether or not her "factions" happen to have happened. "Metaphor", Slater confirms, "is the greatest gift of language, for through it, we can propel ... otherwise wordless experiences into shapes and sounds" (ibid, p. 219). Through *Lying*, Slater finds a way to witness that *something* that unsettles Lauren.

Acting epileptic and speaking lies, however, prove insufficient channels to release Lauren's quaking testimony. Slater cites *mythomania*, the compulsive need to tell stories, as a symptom of her "disease," but she also lists *hypergraphia*, "the driving compulsion to write," as a core element of her illness (ibid, p. 98). In order to witness, *Lying* suggests, Lauren must write. However Eurocentric and logocentric, the centrality of writing to witnessing is critically substantiated. Felman, Laub, Hampl, and Henke all assert that speaking testimony is not sufficient to overcome trauma. In order to heal, one must move beyond orality and physically record one's experience (Felman and Laub 1992, p. 63; Hampl 1999, p. 34; Henke 2001, p. 142). This assertion raises troubling questions for those who cannot write or do not relate to writing as a therapeutic process. Scriptotherapy, however, does resonate with Slater. The moment she realizes she can write her way out of illness, she celebrates: "something happened to me" (Slater 2000, p. 111). "I went straight to ... my notebook. Holding my pen, I wrote faster and faster ... The words were pure pleasure, physical rhythmic objects that released dreams like birds from a magician's fist ... and when I was done, I saw a story before me" (ibid, p. 111). In this scene, rather than seizing, Slater is seized with inspiration. In writing, she discovers not only a story before her but her inner being, released "like birds" from a constricted psychic fist (ibid, p. 111). Writing proves restorative, helping both the author, Slater, and her narrator, Lauren, articulate a painful past.

In *Autobiographics*, Leigh Gilmore critiques autobiography and memoir for inciting authors to construct a falsely unitive "I" (Gilmore 1994, p. ix). Gilmore's view overlooks that life-writing, though necessarily self-absorbed, does not require authors to perform essentialized selves. Autobiography and memoir, Felman attests, can help traumatized persons witness memories, otherwise "overwhelmed by occurrences that have not settled into understanding or remembrance, acts that cannot be ... assimilated into full cognition" (Felman and Laub 1992, p. 5). If Felman is correct, writers such as Slater can use their work to write through shattering experiences. In the preface to *Lying*, Slater makes a similar point through the character of Dr. Hayward Krieger, an expert she invents to define memoir as "a new kind of Heideggerian truth, the truth of the liminal, the not-knowing, the truth of confusion" (Slater 2000, p. x). Rather than underscoring a unified "I", memoirs like Slater's open aporias of "I" and "you." Slater writes: "I am two separate people, just like me and you" (ibid, p. 173). In such passages, Slater does not assign a unitive "I" to her narrator, but instead exposes Lauren's multiple, contradictory selves that crash into and seize away from one another. In witnessing this liminal identity, Slater deconstructs Gilmore's essentialized "I." She also (perhaps unknowingly) underscores the process of dual-witnessing, when a primary witness (or "I") occupies the same psychic or textual space as a secondary witness ("you"), without merging wholly into the other.

The duality inherent in Slater's narrator is complicated further when Lauren acknowledges that she encompasses more than "two separate people"—"me and you" (ibid, p. 173)—but, like Walt Whitman, "contain[s] multitudes" (Whitman 2007, p. 67): "I didn't live [only] as Lauren," Slater writes. "I lived ... as April, Bobby, Maria and Juliette. 'I am an epileptic,' Juliette said. ... 'I have seizures all the time'" (Slater 2000, p. 87). Within the supposedly cohesive genre of memoir, Slater's narrative voice is not unified. Instead, her work witnesses multiplicity—"April," "Bobby," "Maria," and "Juliette," written in both first person ("I am an epileptic") and third person ("Juliette said")—without erasing or diminishing elements of herself. In *Lying*, Slater breaks open the assumed authority of the autobiographical "I" by adding something more—that which Slater perpetually attempts to witness. Lauren explains:

> I'd like to ... lay out the possibilities ... (A) I have epilepsy ... (B) I have epilepsy, but due to ... the need to exaggerate, ... you should believe only selectively what I have recorded here. (C) I don't have epilepsy at all, ... but I do have Munchausen's, and what you have here before you is a true portrait of a ... sick mind under siege ... (D) I have neither Munchausen's nor epilepsy ... but I did grow up with a mother so wedded to denial ... that I became confused about reality and ... fell in love with tall tales. (ibid, p. 161)

In mapping out these possibilities, Slater suggests that A, B, C, or D alone do not characterize Lauren or her condition. Lauren does not "simply" have epilepsy (A). Nor, according to her understanding of metaphoric and psychic truth, does she *not* have epilepsy (D). Rather, identity and experience are located at the intersecting incongruities of A through D: Her "truth" cannot be reduced to a single letter or explanation but is found instead at the juncture of those innumerable, conflicting *somethings* that exist within her, which can never be adequately conveyed. The only way to witness a slippery self, Slater suggests, is to write a slippery memoir. "I became a memoirist," she acknowledges (ibid, p. 144). "What else could I be?" (ibid, p. 144).

In *Lying*, Slater never clearly indicates whether or not Lauren witnesses trauma successfully. As her narrator's writer-arranger, however, Slater does seem able to write across the "A" through "D" factors to witness that she feels traumatized and is not sure why (which represents a kind of trauma in itself). *Lying*, then, speaks not to the factual truth of particular childhood memories (e.g., Lauren's battle with epilepsy and Munchausen's syndrome), but to the memoirist's struggle to witness ineffable experiences. "In this book," she writes, "I have finally, finally been able to tell a tale eluding me for years, a tale I have tried over and over again to utter, the story of my past ... I have told it all [now] and it is relief ... to put it to rest" (ibid, p. 220). Having witnessed her inability to witness, Slater concludes her memoir and affirms that she may now rest, psyche sated.

Where Slater ends, readers begin, a step that unlocks the second element of dual-witnessing: for a writer-narrator to witness primarily, readers must witness her story secondarily. A primary witness may not always know how her testimony is received. Slater, for example, cannot possibly know how each reader responds to *Lying*. One may wonder how dual-witnessing functions in such cases. In answer, I focus on the reception to the text itself. An attention to textual reception should not suggest that an author's experience is somehow less important than her published work. Instead, I argue that a sustained empathic response to both author and text is vital. With reception theorists, such as Stanley Fish (Fish 1970), Wolfgang Iser (Iser 1978), and Louise Rosenblatt (Rosenblatt 1978), I maintain that, while a reader cannot always communicate with an author, one can converse—or dual-witness—with a text. Reader-response critics maintain that reading is not only a passive, but also an active process (Jauss 1982, p. 19; Phelan 1997, p. 227; Goldstein and Machor 2008, p. xiv). When reading, James Phelan explains, "the text acts upon us and we act upon it; the text calls upon—and we respond with—our cognitive, emotive, social, and ethical selves" (Phelan 1997, p. 228). The same, I argue, is true of witnessing, which, like reading, is neither one-sided, nor passive, but dual and active. Thus, while a survivor gains or suffers the most, depending on how her narrative is read, both dual-witnessing and anti-witnessing can take place beyond the purview of a writer-narrator. In such cases, the text itself serves as the primary witness, and the reader continues to function as the secondary witness.

Slater hints at the need to be witnessed secondarily in her use of the first-person plural to witness instances that appear to affect her alone. When speaking about her propensity for falsehood and fascination with epilepsy, for example, she declares: "We"—not I—"create all sorts of lies, all sorts of stories and metaphors. . . . Our stories are seizures. They clutch us, they are spastic grasps, they are losses of consciousness. Epileptics, every one of us; I am not alone" (Slater 2000, p. 197). One could read this statement as proof of Slater's projected hope that some "other" shares her reality. Her assertion also prompts readers to enter into her existence, to embrace her history, however foreign her experiences initially seem, so that writer and reader may collaborate.

Inspiring this dual-witnessing appears to be one of Slater's main goals in *Lying*. In testifying to her trauma, she simultaneously inspires readerly affinity and support. "Understand," she entreats (ibid, p. 84). She then spends the rest of her memoir pushing readers to realize her deceptively simple appeal. As *Lying* progresses, so too does the urgency with which the request to "understand" is presented, so that in detailing "how to market this book" (ibid, p. 159), Slater's need to be witnessed secondarily reads as almost desperate. "I am giving you a portrait of the essence of me", she writes, but "living where I do . . . in the chasm that cuts through thought . . . is lonely" (ibid, p. 163). She thus implores:

> Come with me, reader. Enter the confusion with me. . . . Give up the ground with me, because sometimes that frightening floaty place is really the truest of all. Kierkegaard says, . . . 'We are at our most honest when we are lost.' Enter that lostness with me. Live in the place I am, where the view is murky, where the connecting bridges and orienting maps have been . . . stripped away. . . . Together we will journey. We are disoriented, and all we ever really want is a hand to hold. . . . I am so happy you are holding me in your hands. I am sitting far away from you, but when you turn the pages, I feel a flutter in me, and wings rise up. (ibid, p. 163)

Slater's metaphor—that readers hold her in our hands—is evocative in that we both physically hold her book and—she hopes—choose to hold her act of primary witnessing in our hands, to witness her narrative secondarily.

Although some may contest that *Lying* discourages secondary witnessing (how can we engage what we cannot believe or understand?), the reverse is also true. *Lying*'s mutability actually encourages readerly response: the more aporias written into a text, the more liminal spaces blurred, the more easily a reader can enter a textual conversation. Slater impels this process by placing herself and her reader on the same page, so that we journey together in the same direction. In the passage above, Slater acknowledges: "we are"—not I am—"disoriented" (ibid, p. 163). She confuses us, so that we may enter into, and witness secondarily, her narrator's confusion. By telling her story unreliably, Slater thrusts her readers into an ictal space, enabling us to occupy more than one position at once: that of truth and falsehood, of writer and reader, and of primary and secondary witness. Through entering into Lauren's consciousness, readers situate themselves at a liminal core of multiple, assumed opposites, a shifting, seizing space that offers the opportunity, first, to experience what it feels like to be Lauren and, second, to dual-witness, i.e., to enter into—and witness out of—the psychic space of another, without becoming other.

However many metaphors Slater offers to elucidate her history, she poses an equal number of questions. "Clutch at what?", she queries. "You tell me" (ibid, p. 216). Earlier she queries:

"Is metaphor in memoir, in *life*, an alternate form of honesty or simply an evasion?" (ibid, p. 192). By asking and not answering questions, by refusing to delineate what her trauma is, by acknowledging that she herself does not know the answers to the questions she poses, Slater opens her trauma to her readers. Her metaphors signify that which is unknowable in Lauren's life and prompt readers to examine the unknowable in all of our lives. We fill in her blanks with our own memories (without becoming Slater ourselves). In this way, as Diane Freedman and Olivia Frey write of life-writing in general, *Lying* "hold[s] our attention in ways that more objective, distanced pieces will not" (Freedman and Frey 2004, p. 5). When Slater's primary witnessing is joined by readers' secondary witnessing, the memoir encourages dual-witnessing, whereas texts which more clearly divorce the writer-narrator from the reader-respondent may not.

Slater pushes readers toward dual identification through the use of the second person in the description of her first seizure. "You grit your teeth", she writes. "You clench, a spastic look crawls across your face, your legs thrash like a funky machine, you hit hard and spew, you grind your teeth with such a force that you might wake up with a mouth full of molar dust, tooth ash, the residue of words you've never spoken, but should have" (Slater 2000, p. 19). By writing "you" instead of "I", Slater distances herself from her speaker, depicting a split identity. The dissociation is also inclusive, welcoming the reader into her liminal space.

Lying's trauma, Slater suggests, is not something Lauren must face alone, but something that individual and collective readers—both included in the singular and plural "you"—can and should witness with her. Slater continues her description by shifting between first and second person narration: "You bite your mouth—I do at least—chew it to pieces from the inside out" (ibid, p. 19), as if to suggest that this experience is shared by her readers. Though Slater writes from the particulars of her own experiences, her memoir's content and form both prompt readers to recognize inter-relationality. If one comes away from *Lying* with even a vague sense that *something* has happened during the reading process, the text may witness the *it* Slater writes to work through.

Slater's determination to witness primarily misses its mark when readers refuse to witness her text secondarily. Although the memoir opens the possibility of dual-witnessing, this process can also be hard to effect. Trauma theorist, Cathy Caruth, asserts that "the difficulty" of "responding to traumatic stories in a way that does not lose their impact, that does not reduce them to clichés or turn them all into versions of the same story", is a "problem for therapists and literary critics alike" (Caruth 1995, p. vii). A paradox of *Lying* is that what makes Slater's primary witnessing possible (the use of metaphor to witness truth) can also preclude the reader's ability to witness secondarily. Indeed, Lauren's fabrications so often alienate readers, that her memoir's potential to witness is diminished. Rather than entering into Lauren's psyche, readers sometimes distance themselves from her account, too annoyed that Slater has lied to them to examine why she has lied. This response is natural. Many believe that the only acceptable type of memoir is one that is always "truthful." Autobiographical theorist, Andrea Dworkin, contends that writing is a "sacred trust. It means telling the truth. . . . It means . . . never lying" (Bleich 2004, p. 42). Readers who agree denounce Slater for her falsehoods. In doing so, they may anti-witness her testimony.

Consider, for example, the reviews *Lying* has received on amazon.com.[4] While many praise Slater's text, just as many censure it for its dishonesty. P. Seaton writes: "I couldn't trust the narrator . . . [which] meant also that I was . . . unable to feel close to [her] and really understand her motivations" (amazon.com 2008). Seaton (2008) recognizes that witnessing secondarily—"feel[ing] close to the narrator" and "understand[ing] her motivations"—is an "important role" of memoirs. The reviewer, however, overlooks that Slater includes falsehoods in her text to portray her reality more (not less) accurately and to invite readers into her psyche, not to alienate them from it.

---

4   Amazon.com is not a scholarly or an authoritative source, but its reviews can reflect how general (i.e., non-academic) readers interpret texts.

Tori Albert also dismisses *Lying* on amazon.com because she feels Slater manipulates readers instead of reaching out to them. "As a reader" Albert writes, I felt like a pawn in her self-serving game ('Am I lying to you?'), disappointed and jarred" (Albert 2010). Albert is not alone in this critique. The depiction of Slater as puppeteer is echoed in a *New York Times*' review, in which Janet Malin queries: "If this memoir is merely a feat of gamesmanship, what would induce the reader to play along?" (Malin 2000). Malin's rhetorical question implies that entering Slater's world is a waste of readers' time. If reader-reviewers, however, refuse to "play along" with Slater, they also cannot witness her account secondarily, and *Lying*'s witnessing potential lies dormant.

Slater recognizes this danger and returns repeatedly to the question of who is reading her story, and how. In an interview Lauren submits to her college newspaper (in which she interviews herself), Lauren asks herself: "Is writing one way you have of reaching out to others?" (Slater 2000, p. 173). "Absolutely," she replies (ibid, p. 173). If Slater's writing is rejected by others, if her "reaching out" is refused, her trauma remains un-witnessed. Even when readers assume they know her, Slater is skeptical. She asserts, for instance, that those who "know nothing about my slipperiness," who read her memoir not metaphorically but "quite literally" (ibid, p. 162) fail to witness her secondarily. And when readers refuse to witness secondarily, she cannot witness primarily through *Lying*. "If you read [my memoir] that way," she writes, "I will feel I have failed" (ibid, p. 162). Slater is consumed with being read in the "right" way, with witnessing primarily and being witnessed secondarily. Only then can she write to work through inexpressible trauma.

Slater's fear that she will be misread (or not read at all) is reasonable: *Lying*'s testimony is not often met, and both writer and narrator seem to feel more isolated and rejected (anti-witnessed) than seen, heard, and supported (dual-witnessed). "Lying is lonely," Slater writes. "No one knows you," and "when people are interested in you, you understand it's for false reasons, and you get depressed" (ibid, p. 133). Lauren's writing tutor, Christopher Marin, for example, seduces her by pretending to witness her secondarily, while only using her to satisfy his sex addiction. When teenaged Lauren first meets the adult Marin, she believes she "love[s] him", simply "because I thought he might love me" in return (ibid, p. 125). After sleeping with her teacher, however, Lauren discovers that Marin never actually attempted to witness her secondarily and that "if he ever … knew how … my whole damn being could turn into froth and spasm, I think he would have hated me" (ibid, p. 128). Rather than entering into Lauren's reality, Marin's interaction with his pupil reads more as an example of victimization or anti-witnessing than of mutual connection or dual-witnessing. Legally, sex between a minor (Lauren) and an adult (Marin) constitutes sexual assault. The way Marin treats Lauren reinforces the predatory nature of their supposedly consensual "relationship". The distinction Slater draws between a consensual relationship and an assaultive one parallels the disparity I identify between dual-witnessing and anti-witnessing. Dual-witnessing is a form of intercourse, a "social communication between individuals" (OED 2017b, sense 2a), that, like sex (ibid, sense 2), represents an avenue of intimacy. Those who abuse the intimacy established during dual-witnessing contribute to—versus combat—the trauma of the primary witness's experience.

Indeed, after her experience with Marin, Lauren begins to link perceived acts of anti-witnessing (especially by male authority figures) to sexual assault. When, for example, she tells her counselor at Brandeis that she has epilepsy, that she has undergone operations to be "cured", and that she still finds herself seizing, the counselor dismisses her: "There is no such part of the brain … as the 'temporal amygdalan area.' There is no such thing as … 'eliopathic epilepsy.' … There is no Dr. Neu anywhere in the world who would perform a corpus callostomy on a patient with TLE" (Slater 2000, pp. 175–76). At first Lauren protests, but when her counselor demands to see her scar as "proof" of her testimony, she accuses him of attempting to violate her. "I understood", Slater writes. "He was a pervert. He wanted to touch me. I jerked away" (ibid, p. 177). What seems assaultive to Lauren is not only that a man tried to touch her without consent but that he reached out to her without connecting to her—that, like Marin, he anti-witnessed her when he could have witnessed her secondarily. A dark irony exists in reading "therapist" as "the rapist". Refusal to witness, Slater implies, marks a kind of assault. Believing that her counselor peered into her scarred self without attempting to engage her reality, Lauren reports him to the Brandeis Counseling Center. Slater holds him up as a counter-example to her readers, as if to warn us to engage *Lying* only if we are willing to witness its content secondarily.

The memoir's most evocative example of anti-witnessing is illustrated, not by those who actively mistreat Lauren, but by those who come close to dual-witnessing, only to renounce the connection. Lauren's friends in Alcoholics Anonymous, for example, encourage her to witness primarily, coaxing: "Admitting the truth is the bravest, most healing thing" (ibid, p. 204). When she divulges that "I have never been able to admit or even know the truth. ... It's part of my disease" (ibid, p. 204), Lauren feels as if she may witness for the first time. "I felt the story take shape", she extols, "and it really was true, it flew from me" (ibid, p. 205). She thanks the group for having "given me a way to tell my tale" (ibid, p. 207).

When Lauren tries to share a deeper truth, that she is not an alcoholic but has suffered an unspeakable trauma as the result of a "disease of (ibid, p. 206), her listeners silence her: "Shhh", Brad says (ibid, p. 212). Amy adds: "Too much truth can overwhelm a person" (ibid, p. 212). Rather than dual-witnessing, Lauren's audience anti-witnesses her. To come close to forming a connection only to have the moment taken away unsettles Lauren. "My facts blew away", she recalls, "and I found myself back in the world I knew best, the strange warped world of so many stories—I am an alcoholic I am not an alcoholic; I am an epileptic I am not an epileptic" (ibid, p. 213). Unable to witness primarily, she finds herself isolated in a group, alienated by the loneliness of a trauma that she must—yet cannot—witness. Notably, Lauren attempts in this scene to witness orally. Slater, conversely, witnesses by writing Lauren's testimony down. Trauma and autobiographical critics may argue that Slater is successful where Lauren is not, because Lauren *speaks* her testimony to listeners who are not receptive, versus Slater, who *writes* her narrative for readers who (ideally) receive her text more willingly. While the group at Alcoholics Anonymous shuts down Lauren's attempt to witness, Slater's readers still have the opportunity to contribute to her narrative through witnessing it secondarily.

The succeeding question is "how?". If theorists insist that survivors write through their experiences, in order to heal, what is the ensuing responsibility of the reader to the writer of traumatic testimony? How can we avoid anti-witnessing a work in order to witness its contents secondarily? Slater does not answer these questions directly in *Lying*. She does, however, model dual-witnessing when Lauren listens to another person's testimony at an Alcoholics Anonymous meeting. "The woman took the microphone and lowered her lips to it", Lauren recalls. "Her mouth began to tremble and tears came out, silvering her sad, sad face" (ibid, p. 179). As the other woman speaks, Lauren finds that "then I, too, wanted to cry, because the idea of her unhappiness brings me always to a dark and difficult place" (ibid, p. 179). Lauren has never met this woman before, but when the stranger begins to witness, she connects to her. This scene directly follows Lauren's escape from her counselor's office, from the threat of his anti-witnessing, and Slater is able in this moment to convey what dual-witnessing is: the convergence with another's testimony while still maintaining one's own alterity.

Still, the witnessing Slater evokes is so demanding that even Lauren cannot withstand it. When the speaker who moved Lauren to tears asks her to hear her fifth step—the "admitting to ourselves and to another human being the exact nature of our wrongs" (itself a kind of dual-witnessing)—Lauren "grow[s] bored" and disengages (ibid, p. 194). Such scenes underscore dual-witnessing's difficulty, even as *Lying* underscores its necessity. Witnessing, Slater suggests, is nearly impossible both to begin and to sustain—for writer-narrators and reader-respondents alike.

Readers are called to dual-witness nevertheless. Freedman and Frey emphasize that "we cannot stand outside these discussions, dispassionate, untouched, neither as readers nor as writers" (Freedman and Frey 2004, p. 5). Instead of anti-witnessing traumatic truths, we must challenge ourselves to engage traumatic testimony as secondary witnesses. Slater acknowledges that what readers do with *Lying*, what we take from its substance, is up to us: The choice, she reminds us, is ultimately "in [our] hands" (Slater 2000, p. 139). Slater writes *Lying* to witness enigmatic traumas. Whether or not her project is successful depends largely on readers' parallel (in)ability to dual-witness. Despite *Lying*'s orchestrated moments of confusion and confabulation, then, its overarching message is in fact quite clear: readers should not disavow Slater's narrative because it is difficult to believe or to understand. We are incited instead to enter into *Lying* actively and to witness its "factions" secondarily, so that, together, we can let seizing truths lie.

Conflicts of Interest: The author declares no conflict of interest.

References

Albert, Tori. 2010. "Loved the First $\frac{1}{4}$". April 8. Available online: https://smile.amazon.com/Lying-Metaphorical-Memoir-Lauren-Slater/dp/014200006X/ref=cm_cr_arp_d_product_top?ie=UTF8 (accessed on 5 November 2010).

Allison, Dorothy. 1996. *Two or Three Things I Know for Sure*. New York: Penguin Books.

Bleich, David. 2004. Finding the Right Word: Self-Inclusion and Self-Inscription. In *Autobiographical Writing across the Disciplines: A Reader*. Edited by Diane Freedman and Olivia Frey. Durham: Duke University Press, pp. 41–67.

Brison, Susan. 2003. *Aftermath: Violence and the Remaking of a Self*. Princeton: Princeton University Press.

Cathy Caruth, ed. 1995. *Trauma: Explorations in Memory*. Baltimore: Johns Hopkins University Press.

Chun, Wendy Hui Kyong. 2002. Unbearable Witness: Toward a Politics of Listening. In *Extremities: Trauma, Testimony, and Community*. Edited by Nancy Miller and Jason Tougaw. Urbana: University of Illinois Press, pp. 143–65.

Craps, Stef. 2013. *Postcolonial Witnessing: Trauma out of Bounds*. Houndmills: Palgrave Macmillan.

Ellerby, Janet. 2001. *Intimate Reading: The Contemporary Women's Memoir*. Syracuse: Syracuse University Press.

Farrell, Kirby. 1998. *Post-Traumatic Culture: Injury and Interpretation in the Nineties*. Baltimore: Johns Hopkins University Press.

Felman, Shoshana, and Dori Laub. 1992. *Testimony: Crises of Witnessing in Literature, Psychoanalysis, and History*. New York: Routledge Press.

Fish, Stanley. 1970. Literature in the Reader: Affective Stylistics. *New Literary History* 2: 123–62. [CrossRef]

Freedman, Diane, and Olivia Frey. 2004. Introduction. In *Autobiographical Writing Across the Disciplines: A Reader*. Edited by Diane Freedman and Olivia Frey. Durham: Duke University Press, pp. 1–40.

Gilmore, Leigh. 1994. *Autobiographics: A Feminist Theory of Women's Self-Representation*. Ithaca: Cornell University Press.

Goldstein, Philip, and James Machor. 2008. Introduction: Reception Study. Achievements and New Directions. In *New Directions in American Reception Study*. Edited by Philip Goldstein and James Machor. Oxford: Oxford University Press, pp. xi–xxviii.

Hampl, Patricia. 1999. *I Could Tell You Stories: Sojourns in the Lands of Memory*. New York: W.W. Norton & Co.

Henke, Suzette. 2001. *Shattered Subjects: Trauma and Testimony in Women's Life-Writing*. New York: St. Martin's Press.

Herman, Judith. 1997. *Trauma and Recovery: The Aftermath of Violence—From Domestic Abuse to Political Terror*. New York: Basic Books.

Iser, Wolfgang. 1978. *The Act of Reading: A Theory of Aesthetic Response*. Baltimore: Johns Hopkins University Press.

Jauss, Hans Robert. 1982. *Toward an Aesthetic of Reception*. Translated by Timothy Bahti. Minneapolis: University of Minnesota Press.

Linton, Simi. 1998. *Claiming Disability Knowledge and Identity*. New York: New York University Press.

Malin, Janet. 2000. Book of the Times: It Could Be Fact or Fiction . . . or Something Else. *The New York Times*. June 22. Available online: https://partners.nytimes.com/library/books/062200slater-book-review.html (accessed on 5 November 2010).

Miller, Nancy K., and Jason Tougaw. 2002. Introduction. In *Extremities: Trauma, Testimony, and Community*. Edited by Nancy Miller and Jason Tougaw. Urbana: University of Illinois Press, pp. 1–25.

OED. 2017a. Epilepsy. Oxford English Dictionary Online. Available online: http://public.oed.com/?post_type=page&s=epilepsy (accessed on 18 September 2010).

OED. 2017b. Intercourse. Oxford English Dictionary Online. Available online: http://public.oed.com/?post_type=page&s=intercourse (accessed on 18 October 2017).

OED. 2017c. Witness. 2017. Oxford English Dictionary Online. Available online: http://public.oed.com/?post_type=page&s=witness (accessed on 18 October 2017).

Phelan, James. 1997. Toward a Rhetorical Reader-Response Criticism: The Difficult, the Stubborn, and the Ending of *Beloved*. In *Toni Morrison: Critical and Theoretical Approaches*. Edited by Nancy Peterson. Baltimore: Johns Hopkins University Press, pp. 225–44.

Rosenblatt, Louise. 1978. *The Reader, the Text, the Poem: The Transactional Theory of the Literary Work*. Carbondale: Southern Illinois University Press.

Rothberg, Michael. 2009. *Multidirectional Memory: Remembering the Holocaust in the Age of Decolonization*. Stanford: Stanford University Press.

Seaton, P. 2008. Well Done But Not Fascinating Enough. October 8. Available online: https://smile.amazon.com/Lying-Metaphorical-Memoir-Lauren-Slater/dp/014200006X/ref=cm_cr_arp_d_product_top?ie=UTF8 (accessed on 5 November 2010).

Slater, Lauren. 2000. *Lying*. New York: Penguin.

Whitman, Walt. 2007. *Leaves of Grass*. New York: Dover Publications, Inc., First published 1855.

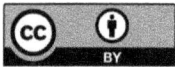

humanities

MDPI

Article

World-Hating: Apocalypse and Trauma in *We Need to Talk about Kevin*

Sean Desilets

Departments of Film Studies, English, and Gender Studies, Westminster College, Salt Lake City, UT 84111, USA;
sdesilets@westminstercollege.edu

Received: 19 September 2017; Accepted: 6 November 2017; Published: 13 November 2017

Abstract: Lynne Ramsay's 2011 film *We Need to Talk about Kevin* alternates between two narrative times, one occurring before its protagonist Eva's son commits a terrible crime, and one after. The film invites us to read the crime as a traumatic event in Eva's life, an event of such terrible force that it transforms Eva's identity. This essay uses Jacob Taubes's understanding of Gnosticism to suggest that this event does not transform who Eva is, but rather how she knows. Like a Gnostic believer, Eva comes to understanding the fundamental ontological evil of community life. Eva's 'trauma,' her alienation from the world she occupies, predates Kevin's crime, but the aftermath of that crime reveals her alienation to her. The worldview thus presented by the film casts some light on how art house films are marketed. Like many middlebrow products, art house films present marketers with the challenge of concealing the fact that the commodity they are selling is indeed a commodity. This ambivalent distrust of the marketplace is a softened repetition of the Gnostic's anticosmism, and *We Need to Talk About Kevin* both performs and thematizes a displacement from the world that is primary, not contingent upon any traumatic event.

Keywords: *We Need to Talk about Kevin*; Lynne Ramsay; Gnosticism; trauma; independent cinema; marketing; Jacob Taubes

---

'Trauma' is a recent entry in a long series of concepts that seek to name a curious element of Western experience: what places us in the world (call it 'nature' or 'reality') seems paradoxically coterminous with what *dis*places us from it. This mirroring connection between placement and displacement derives from the human tendency to (mis)take ourselves to be radically different from everything else that exists. Two related factors distinguish the concept of trauma from other concepts directed at this problem (for instance, 'alienation' and 'neurosis'): the concept of trauma places special emphasis on temporality, and, in its psychological interiorization, it frankly acknowledges the coincidence of placement and displacement as the temporal locus of identity. Trauma is always a matter of memory or its failure, and as such, always stages a confrontation between present and past. For trauma, this moment of turning back to the past is the pivot upon which selfhood hangs. Trauma itself occurs in a paradoxical temporality; its pivotal character means it is decisively in the past even as its role as the basis of traumatized identity keeps it in the present as long as that identity exists. Meanwhile trauma, because it generates new identities for its victims out of material that intrudes from the outside, also forces us to recognize that identity itself is dependent upon the world from which it seeks to disentangle itself. In Freud's model, for instance, what makes trauma traumatic is the process by which external stimuli install themselves (or their psychic representatives) inside the borders that the psyche uses to protect itself from external threats (Freud 1961, pp. 35–36).

My description subordinates trauma to what I take to be a more persistent, even foundational problem: the coterminous quality of the placement and displacement. That way of conceiving trauma will be important to me because although I will be approaching a film *about* trauma, my means of approach will seem at first glance far removed from the affective frenzy that we associate with traumatic experiences. My reading of this film, Lynne Ramsay's *We Need to Talk About Kevin* (2011, henceforth shortened to *Kevin*), can be understood as an effort to justify this conceptual hierarchy in which displacement precedes trauma.[1] *We Need to Talk about Kevin*'s protagonist experiences profound social displacement that seems to originate in a traumatic event, albeit one that culminates a long traumatic period. The film reveals that the displacement actually precedes the event, both temporally and logically. Just as importantly, the film's ambivalent participation in the cinematic marketplace marks its self-consciousness about the (as it were) traumatic effect of commodity status on artworks. In this, it is not different from most other art house films, which must approach their self-presentation as commodities gingerly because their very appeal *as* commodities includes a certain distrust of the mass-media marketplace (Newman 2009, p. 17). This essay begins by addressing the question of how *Kevin* presents itself to its audience and how that mode of address relates to the history of art cinema consumption in the US. It next turns to the text of the film itself, extracting from it a kind of explanation or allegorization of the logic behind this mode of address. I will read the film as a contemporary repetition of a very old and especially elaborate confrontation with the simultaneity of placement and displacement: the second-century phenomenon of Gnosticism—particularly as described by twentieth-century theologian Jacob Taubes. The upshot of this analysis will be an argument that the text of *Kevin* amounts to a version of the gnostic 'insight' that the properly initiated can read the signs of the world's foundational perfidy in the texture of the world itself, and that the reading of these signs presents the possibility of escape, even if it is only escape from delusion and not from the underlying misery of living in the world. My aim is to present Gnosticism as a moment in the genealogy of trauma, using it to excavate the links between the ambivalent marketing of arthouse films and this film's way of representing traumatized subjectivity.

1. Commodity–Trauma

The marketing of American art films may seem at first like a somewhat cold precinct in which to seek out the origins of trauma. But marketing is always a matter of exploiting consumers' fears and desires. In the case of the marketing of independent art house films, the trauma to be feared is the condition of being either a commodity or its consumer. Like many middlebrow products, indie films present marketers with the challenge of concealing the fact that the commodity they are selling is indeed a commodity. This mandate derives, of course, from the mistaken impression that art and commerce are at odds with one another, an impression that persists in the face of the perfectly obvious fact that most of our artistic experiences come to us directly from markets and cost money. Acknowledging that artworks are also commodities sits uncomfortably for us because we don't *feel* like consumers when we consume artworks. We approach them as means to understand and direct our aspirations, fears, and desires. People who seek out films like *Kevin*, which is adapted from a celebrated contemporary novel and which stars an actor (Tilda Swinton) whose career began in the films of the truly independent director Derek Jarman, do so at least in part because we believe such films to be directed at socially or culturally important problems. These problems are not the ones that are faced by marketers trying to sell commodities to large aggregates of people, and we thus hold to the belief that the primary authors of these films are artists and not marketers. These considerations help explain why the term 'independent' is still used to describe films whose engagement with multinational entertainment corporations is a necessary condition of their availability to the audiences they seek (Tzioumakis 2012, p. 139). The economic trajectory of the American art house marketplace has been well-documented, and its most pertinent feature has been massive participation by 'classics'

---

[1] *Kevin* is one of a series of apocalyptic genre-hybrid thrillers released into the American art house marketplace in 2011, alongside Jeff Nichols's *Take Shelter* (2011), Sean Durkin's *Martha Marcy May Marlene* (2011), and Zal Batmanglij's *The Sound of My Voice* (2011), and Mike Cahill's *Another Earth* (2011). For an assessment of how *Take Shelter* and *Martha Marcy May Marlene* also participate in the dynamic delineated here, see the chapter "Weak Apocalypticism," in my *Hermeneutic Humility and the Political Theology of Cinema: Blind Paul* (Desilets 2017). This essay represents an evolution in my reading of *We Need to Talk about Kevin* in that it places the film's Gnostic sensibility in dialog with its marketing.

divisions of the major Hollywood studios, along with a few commercially-minded and well-capitalized production and/or distribution companies like Miramax. *Kevin's* case is somewhat complicated by the fact that it is not 'American,' though it is set in the US and was aggressively distributed there (by Oscilloscope Laboratories, an independent distributer founded by Adam Yauch of the Beastie Boys, a visitor from another realm in which the term 'independent' aims at a mobile target). Here is how the Hollywood News (2010) described *Kevin's* financing: "Presented by BBC Films and the UK Film Council in association with Footprint Investments LLP, Caemhan Partnership LLP and Lipsync Productions, the film is an Independent/Jennifer Fox production in association with Artina Films and Forward Films." This language deliberately obscures what financial contributions each of these entities made to the film's $7 million budget, but it seems safe to say that much of the film's financing came from British public sources (BBC Films and the UK Film Council). Every other entity listed here clearly hoped to turn a profit on the film (*Kevin* is Oscilloscope's third highest-grossing title ever and Artina's second, although its box office gross of $10 million represents a relatively modest return on investment, and less than $2 million of that came from US ticket sales).[2] In any event, the film's aesthetic reflects its imbrication in a robust corporate film distribution and production system: it generally displays a continuity style calculated not to alienate filmgoers, although the narrative structure is unusually complex and Tilda Swinton's performance is stylized enough to stand out.

The status anxiety that informs the film's marketing comes out most strongly in its presentation of its lurid subject matter. In the 'indiewood' era, the relationship between art cinema and genre cinema has been complex (King 2005, p. 165). Much of the groundwork for American independent cinema's production practices was laid by horror and exploitation filmmakers like Roger Corman, George Romero, and Wes Craven (Sexton 2012, p. 68). Even now, the 'mainstream' American films that are most likely to resemble American independent cinema in terms of budget and production processes are horror films. But because independent films must market themselves as works of art, and because critics wish to speak of these films that way, the genetic and industrial similarities between genre and art house films sometimes escape notice. Seeing the resonance between art house and genre production, and also the pitfalls of too close an association between them, most of the major studios developed and some still maintain separately-branded subsidiaries for genre and art house films (Sexton 2012, p. 81). These marketing maneuvers seem entirely sensible in light of some critical responses to *We Need to Talk about Kevin*. Even before the film was made, Lionel Shriver, the author of the novel upon which is based, expressed concern that the film would fail to do justice to the complexity of the novel's narrative (which is communicated in letters from the protagonist to her ex-husband) and instead play up the 'thriller' elements of the plot (Arendt 2006). Sure enough, several negative reviews purport to see through the film's gloss and find the bad genre film underneath. For Richard Brody in *The New Yorker, We Need to Talk about Kevin* "masquerades as a psychological puzzle but is essentially a horror film full of decorous sensationalism" (Brody 2012, p. 15). Similarly, David Thomson, detecting holes in what he takes to be the film's social realism, complains that "what seems like an attempt to deal with a real problem in child development topples over into being a horror film. Kevin gets far too close to *The Bad Seed* or Damien in *The Omen* for comfort and plausibility" (Thomson 2012). Behind all three of these reservations lies a valuation of psychological insight, which is associated with aesthetic value, over genre tropes, which are associated with shallow commerce. Whether these criticisms strike home or not, the film itself shares their assumptions. It belongs to a time-honored tradition in art house cinema of engaging sensational topics that might lend themselves to genre treatment, but approaching these topics using aesthetic and thematic resources that align better with the demand for psychological realism and social pertinence that are reflected in the critical assessments I refer to above (Tzioumakis 2012, pp. 11–12). That *Kevin* did well critically overall suggests that it was more or less successful in

---

[2]   This information comes from the websites (Box Office Mojo 2017) and The Numbers: Where Data and the Movie Business Meet (The Numbers 2017).

this endeavor. The film meticulously eschews genre elements. There are virtually no scenes of violence, no chases or 'jump scares,' little use of suspense except for one sequence late in the film whose payoff is at least as coldly ironic as it is horrific. In place of genre-associated formal elements, *Kevin* offers a complex narrative structure, a tendency to favor symmetrical and distant framing over expressionist ones, and a resolutely understated performance style. Even Ezra Miller's performance of Kevin is quite retrained, although he manages to give his character a certain glowering menace. Tilda Swinton's performance *is* stylized, but it is so strongly rooted in Eva's frayed psyche that its higher volume seems entirely appropriate. It is not all that surprising that even as David Thomson compares the film to *The Omen*, one feminist scholar has linked it to Chantal Akerman's *Jeanne Dielman, 23 Commerce Quay, 1080 Brussels*, a masterwork of feminist realism (Thornham 2013, pp. 4–5).

Still, these dissenting voices indicate that *We Need to Talk about Kevin* sits uncomfortably in an art house marketplace that challenges directors and producers to appeal to consumers without appearing to appeal to them. This problem stands out especially when one element of a film's public profile resembles the appeal of films that are less shy about their status as commodity objects. *Kevin's* sensational subject matter threatens to make its status as a commodity too visible. To ward off that threat, the film offers aesthetic elements: an elaborate narrative structure, meticulous pacing, and nuanced performances. As Thomson's complaints indicate, critics and audiences also expect psychological and social realism in films of this sort (again, in contrast to the sensationalism of genre films). Trauma often plays a key role in facilitating this kind of realism. The psychological ticks and evasions associated with repression provide opportunities for actors to grant their characters psychological realism (think of Michael Shannon or Jessica Chastain), and the symbolic displacements that surround traumatic historical events often lend such narratives political gravity (as in the films responding to the dirty wars that prevailed in Latin America through the seventies and eighties).[3] In the next section, I will argue that even as *Kevin* gestures at this kind of realism, it also invites an alternative reading that casts the film's commodity-status in a different light.

2. Gnosticism and the Time of Trauma

These two images appear very early in *We Need to Talk about Kevin*. The shot of the white curtain (Figure 1) is the film's first. Two sounds accompany it: that of a domestic sprinkler with its characteristic cadence at first, and then crowd noises layered over the sprinkler. That latter sound turns out to be a bridge to a series of images (including Figure 2 here) depicting the film's protagonist, Eva, as she participates in the La Tomatina festivities in Valencia, Spain. The curtain veils a threshold that runs through the film—the threshold between its two narrative temporalities. The film cuts between these two timeframes; one occurs before Eva passes through the curtain (and ends when she does so) and the other documents her life after she has passed through it. The juxtaposition of these two images at the start of the film compounds these temporalities, as the scene at the Tomatina festival is actually the temporally earliest part of the pre-curtain segment of the film. Following the curtain with the festival suggests that the curtain gives on to this image of Eva, soaked in the flesh of tomatoes, held aloft by her fellow revelers. If the scene at the festival followed the curtain shot in the diegesis, *We Need to Talk about Kevin* would be a very different film. In this shot from the tomato festival, sociality is erotically charged. Eva delights in the press of bodies, slipping against one another and collapsing into a single monochrome mass of limbs and faces. But the relationship between these two images turns out to be excruciatingly ironic. In fact, on the other side of this curtain for Eva is not an experience of orgiastic social participation, but one of total alienation. The actual post-curtain Eva trudges through her miserable, lonely life in the film's present, and everything that takes place before the curtain event is presented in flashbacks. Eva can only remember, painfully, what has been lost at the threshold of

---

3 These films include Luis Puenzo's *La historia oficial/The Official Story* (1985, Argentina), Bruno Barretos' *O Que E Isso, Companheiro?* (1997, Brazil), and Lucrecia Martel's *La mujer sin Cabeza* (2008, Argentina).

the curtain, which is the film's image for the proximity of traumatic experience. I will suggest that something was gained there, too, and that figuring out the relationship between what has been lost and what gained in Eva's passage through the curtain is the real key to understanding the film both as a text and as a commodity. It turns out that the loss and gain are the same thing: Eva loses her connection to other people as she comes to recognize that the social world around her is pervasively vicious and hateful—an understanding from which she has been shielded by her relationship with her repugnant son, Kevin.

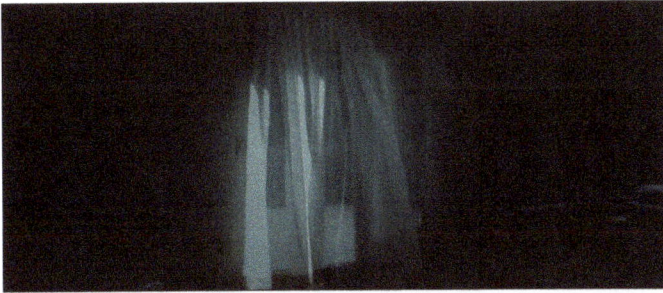

Figure 1. The White Curtain.

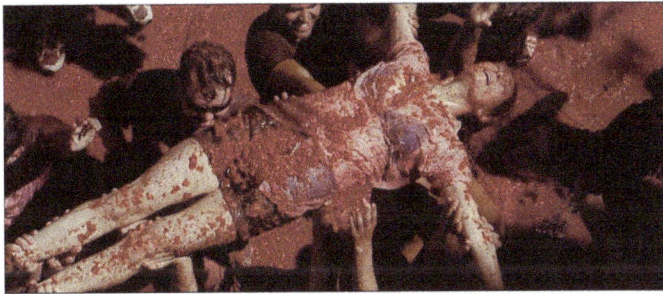

Figure 2. Eva at the La Tomatina festivities.

As I have noted, the narrative is organized around two temporalities, and they meet when the film returns to this curtain image late in its running time. The stark separation between these two temporalities, and their organization around a single pivotal event, suggest that although Eva has lived through a long period of trauma before the event associated with the curtain, this event is uniquely and decisively wounding. The reason, as we will see, is that this event shifts the identity of Eva's tormentor in such a way that previously *private* trauma becomes spectacularly public. In the film's present, its protagonist Eva lives in an unpleasant suburban community that seems particularly hostile to her. Her house and car are routinely vandalized, and her coworkers at a small travel agency either bully or condescend to her. Eva herself appears deeply traumatized. She endures her various humiliations with trembling deference, although she does stubbornly clean up after each incident of vandalism. In the shelter of her home, she drinks heavily and joylessly, eats mechanically, and startles at any sound that intrudes from the outside. Not much happens in this present-tense portion of the film, and everything that does happen (including her rare encounters with decent people) is designed to illustrate Eva's isolation. The narratively valuable events of the film are presented in flashbacks concerning Eva's difficult relationship with Kevin. These flashbacks document Kevin's conception and the entirety of his childhood. He seems to be a sociopath from birth, but his malignity manifests itself especially in his treatment of Eva, to whom he is relentlessly vicious. Kevin also immiserates Eva in less direct ways. In this earlier phase of her life, Eva has been a successful and somewhat glamorous travel writer. Motherhood keeps her from travelling and forces her to work less. The family lives in Manhattan, which clearly accords with Eva's tastes, until Eva's husband Franklin convinces Eva to move to the suburbs on the grounds that it is a better place to raise children (the couple soon after has a second, much nicer, child named Celia). This is the same suburban community that torments Eva in the film's present.

The final sequence in the temporally earlier part of the narrative involves the image of this curtain. It occurs very late in the film, when it finally reveals the events that link the two narrative strains. Eva comes home after having learned that Kevin has massacred several of his classmates during a high school assembly. She enters the house, calls out for her daughter and husband, and gets no response. She approaches the curtain, which hangs in front of a door leading to the family's spacious back yard. As she passes the curtain, the sprinkler's sound, suddenly a bit like laughter, accompanies a tableau depicting the arrow-pierced bodies of Eva's husband Franklin and daughter Celia, lying in the yard; Kevin has murdered them, too. This day robs Eva of whatever sense of affective connection might have been available to her. Two of her family members are dead, and she is isolated from the one that remains both by his own actions and by his imprisonment.

Given all this, it may seem a bit perverse to claim that Eva gains anything when she passes through this white curtain. To get at what I think she *does* gain, I suggest that the film operates under a logic that owes a great deal to the second-century heretical tendency known as Gnosticism. Considerable scholarly attention has been directed at two ways in which Gnosticism influences modernity. The first (less interesting to us) is that the development of orthodox Christianity occurred in part as a response to Gnosticism.[4] The second is that Gnosticism's assiduous cultivation of what we would call a hermeneutics of suspicion about the nature of the manifest world finds echoes in—and probably indirectly influenced—much post-enlightenment philosophy, psychology, and political theory.[5] *We Need to Talk about Kevin* takes this skepticism to the extreme by suggesting that the social world in general is not only valueless but also pernicious. Under this understanding, existence in the social world is itself traumatic.

The more proximate cultural narrative informing *We Need to Talk about Kevin* is the narrative about trauma as a decisive pivot point in human experience. The film's narrative structure suggests an eventual understanding of trauma, under which time is split between two distinct ways of being embodied—unwounded, then wounded. But trauma itself undoes this narrative economy of before and after. It denies the priority of the unwounded body by knotting subjectivity to the moment of wounding. Gnosticism acknowledges this collapsed temporality of trauma. For the Gnostic, embodiment *itself* is conceived as trauma, independent of whatever might happen to a body once it finds itself on earth. There is no such thing as pre-traumatic embodiment.

For purposes of this discussion, I will borrow twentieth-century theologian Jacob Taubes' notion of Gnosticism, which emphasizes some elements of this complex phenomenon over others in an effort to understand how Gnosticism ramifies in modernity. Gnostic systems account for the presence of evil in the world by adducing a radical split between the demiurge who created the cosmos and a transcendent deity that has little or nothing to do with it. The world created by the demiurge not only *contains* evil, it is itself evil, or at least degenerate, because it is the product of a faulty deity. This false God's own existence is usually accounted for in Christian Gnosticism by way of allegorical interpretations of Hebrew scripture that imagine the Hebrew creator God falling away from the true

---

[4] As Kurt Rudolph pointed out, several of the founders of the Christian church wrote heresiological texts against the Gnostics (Rudolph 1987, p. 9).

[5] Ferdinand Christian Bauer makes this case in his 1835 *Die Christliche Gnosis*, and the tradition continues through the work of Jacob Taubes, whom I discuss in greater detail below (Taubes 2010, p. 137).

transcendent God whose only visible manifestation on Earth is Christ's mission.[6] The created cosmos is the product of this false God. It is a terrible error at best, and an obscene blasphemy at worst.

One understands why the Gnostics might think that involvement in this ill-conceived world would be traumatic. They saw themselves as emanations of the true, transcendent God, trapped in material bodies as a consequence of whatever disaster resulted in the creation of the world. They were "Gnostics" exactly because they knew this state of affairs in broad outlines. The true work of Gnosticism was to penetrate the details of the great cosmic conspiracy, a complex web of feints, errors, and allegorical tricks that were secreted away in the Hebrew scriptures and other texts. Discovering the secrets of the fallen world was the path out of it, the path out of the degrading trap of embodiment.

Taubes stresses, however, that the path *out* of the degraded world is the path *in* to the Gnostic's soul (Taubes 2010, p. 102). Given that Gnosticism emerged in the second century, it is startling how thoroughly it addresses itself to *a subject* in a nearly modern sense of the word (Gold 2006, p. 151). Gnosticism anticipates both the epistemological uncertainty and the internalization that typify modern subjectivity. For Taubes, it also maps out the relationship between refusal of the world and historical disappointments. Here is one core element of Taubes's unique reading of Gnostic phenomena: it combines anticosmism with interiorization, and links both to a turning away from history. Taubes sees Gnosticism as "one of the ways in which Jewish and Christian groups react to the deferral of the *parousia*: the accent shifts from the cosmic and historical *parousia* to the entry of the divine into the individual soul. With the decoding of subjectivity, the scene is prepared for Gnostic mythology" (Taubes 2010, p. 73). Thus internalization represents an evasion of historical reality in two senses. First, earthly matters are all lumped together and turned away from in a radical privatization, for lack of a less anachronistic term (this is also in some senses a rejection of community itself; see (O'Regan 2001, p. 33)). Second, time itself ceases to unspool in its unpredictable historical way. When the apocalyptic process moves inside the mystic, it also becomes at least potentially synchronic: "[t]he historical schema of apocalypticism implodes with the disillusion about any predictions of the end of times and retreats inward" (Taubes 2010, p. 74). Instead of moving through time toward an apocalyptic telos (which has proven disappointing in not yielding the hoped-for revelation), the Gnostic moves through an interiorized *space* conceived as *already containing* the transcendence that has been lost in creation. That space is reached by means of what Taubes calls the 'decoding of subjectivity,' which is to say by unraveling the tricks by which the pneumatic spark that constitutes the Gnostic's true identity is locked away in the body and in the material world. Gnosticism ends in an understanding according to which the believer must overcome the forces keeping her apart from God using Gnostic ritual practice and (self-)interpretation (Taubes 2010, p. 68). The Gnostic thus turns ever more inward, in quest of the core of divinity that is buried in the filth of her body.

We Need to Talk about Kevin obviously *does* posit a traumatic moment that occurs during Eva's life. It posits many, in fact, and makes one the sole motive for its disjointed narrative. It thus may not seem to correspond to the model of trauma that I have associated with Gnosticism. The film's narrative structure, though, suggests another reading. After all, we do not know what has so decisively traumatized Eva until the film's conclusion, and up to that point what we get is a clear illustration that while Eva's trauma may have reached its crescendo in the grisly scene in her back yard, it really has a much longer trajectory that corresponds at the very least with Kevin's entire life. Just a little pressure on these two narrative strains reveals a network of connection that belies any simple before-and-after narrative—in other words, the film's narrative logic does not correspond to the reconstruction of events that it invites us to enact once it reaches the decisive threshold of the white curtain.

The most crucial connection between the 'before and after' of the white curtain is Eva's misery. The apparent difference between them is that on the before side Kevin ruins Eva's life, whereas on

---

[6]   These details will be found in one form or another in any account of Gnosticism. I draw primarily from (Rudolph 1987, pp. 53–275).

the after side the neighbors and coworkers that constitute her new social world do so. There are various ways in which these two persecutors are opposed to one another. Most importantly, the community's treatment of Eva is entirely explicable, if ungenerous. In fact, the petty, dreary, nature of the community's treatment of Eva is a feature of the film's social realism—along with the ostentatious acts of vandalism, she suffers minor slights, sideways glances, and little acts of everyday meanness. Kevin appears to represent a break from the film's meticulous psychosocial realism. His evil looks ontological, not socially determined. It emerges in his infancy and expands from there, despite the affluence of Kevin's family and the assiduousness of Eva and Franklin's parenting. The film emphasizes how thoroughly without explanation Kevin's malignancy is. The elements of his identity that *are* socially determined—his fashionability, his critical intelligence—only serve to accentuate the thing about him that is absolute: his fundamental nastiness and brutality. Kevin's anti-sociality goes beyond himself: it also isolates Eva from the social world that is supposed to have provided her with such pleasure in the past—a past visualized in the film exclusively by the scene at the tomato festival (and thus a resolutely mythical past). As her role as Kevin's mother increasingly monopolizes her life, Eva stops working, moves to the suburbs, and loses touch with her publishing contacts. Probably the most excruciating expression of the demoralizing isolation that Kevin imposes on Eva is a scene that takes place before the family has left the city. In it, Eva obtains temporary relief from infant Kevin's incessant crying by pausing near a loud construction site during a walk. Here the tension between the call of the public and the cage of the private, and their analeptic entanglement, find comical but telling expression. Kevin's childhood slowly closes Eva off from the social world. His adolescent act of orgiastic violence—surely an analog to the orgiastic quality of the tomato festival—concludes that trajectory without radically breaking from it.

Kevin's ontological evil, then, is a hostility to the social. Its function is to peel Eva away from the social world she values, and his hatred of that world is comprehensible in terms of the role he plays in Eva's life. It looks like Eva represents—if only in the form of nostalgia—a valuing of sociality, whereas Kevin denigrates sociality at every turn. But the film reveals the inextricability of Eva's and Kevin's attitudes in its two presentations of the white curtain. In the first, it juxtaposes the sound of the suburban sprinkler system in Eva's yard with the dull roar of the Valencian carnival. In the second, it reveals that what really awaits behind the curtain is a vastly darker tableau of ecstatic violation. Kevin's murderous rampage does not represent a break between two phases of Eva's experience. It instead reveals that the bucolic experience of the festival is coterminous not only with the ruthless limiting of Eva's life that results from her submission to heterosexual reproductive normativity, but also with the wretched life that she must live in the aftermath of Kevin's massacre. That Kevin kills *both* his classmates *and* his family is the last of his many acute social observations: the social world and the domestic world are not isolated from one another, but folded together in a network of meanness whose effect on Eva's life has no prehistory.[7] The trauma of the curtain does not thrust Eva into a new way of living, primarily; it thrusts her into a new way of knowing.

Trauma is often conceived as a way of *not* knowing, as a point at which the epistemological resources of the human mind break down. As Cathy Caruth puts it, "trauma is not locatable in the simple violent or original event in an individual's past, but rather in the way that its very unassimilated nature—the way it is precisely *not known* in the first instance—returns to haunt the survivor later on" (Caruth 1996, p. 4). Gnostic anti-cosmism spreads traumatic non-knowledge across all manifest perceptions of the world. To see the manifest world is to look away from the only knowledge it can provide, the knowledge of its own profound degradation. On the other hand, Gnosticism offers that knowledge, terrible though it may be, as a genuine and absolute truth whose understanding is also a

---

[7] The novel from which *Kevin* is adapted does not forge this link between the family and the broader society. Though the details are not entirely clear, the reader knows that Kevin has committed a massacre from early in the book. But Franklin and Celia's deaths comes as a surprise because the narrative is communicated in letters from Eva to Franklin, letters that suggest a continuing though estranged relationship between them (see Shriver 2003).

reversal of the traumatic wound that is existence itself. The knowledge of the Gnostic is structurally opposed to the knowledge of the manifest world, just as its content is a virulent disgust *at* that world.

Indeed, Eva learns that the social world she confronts in the absence of her family justifies Kevin's hatred of it. The collective virtually steps into the place left behind by Kevin's incarceration, continuing his merciless and arbitrary cruelty toward Eva—but taking away the alibi that Kevin himself represented in his inexplicable and aberrant asociality. The film's narrative thus depicts not a radical, traumatic break in Eva's experience, but rather the gradual convergence of the ontological evil represented by Kevin and the petty social evil represented by the community. They meet at the resolution of the parallel narrative lines, in the confluence of Kevin's massacre at the high school and Eva's discovery of the scene at home. The conclusion toward which the narrative moves, then, is that social evil and ontological evil are identical. Kevin's acts of violence amount to a chiasmic crossing of private and public, a hyperbolic airing of the family's dirty laundry that also marks itself as a revelation of the social world's dirty secret. The film offers a grotesque parody of the social-psychological claim that violent acts are socially determined. For *Kevin*, the social world is the proper home of the ontological evil that seems to reside in private individuals, and the relation between the two is not causal but synecdochic. This film is not at all a work of social realism in the traditional sense of the word, but rather a dark parody of realism that posits evil as inexplicable and pervasive.

In discovering the truth, Eva reenacts the Gnostic's journey, and the film thus illustrates certain features of Gnosticism that persist in contemporary western culture. Taubes indicates that Gnosticism emerges from disappointed messianic hopes. It takes only a glance at our shot of Eva held aloft by her companions in Valencia to see that Eva's social desires are at least iconographically messianic. Taubes also says that Gnostic anticosmism redirects myth in two ways: relocating it *inside* the Gnostic subject and synchronizing the telos of the soteriological trajectory of Judeo-Christian monotheism in the form of an emerging (self-)knowledge (Taubes 2010, p. 74). This film's narrative structure shows that the turning-inward of Eva's identity, which is easily misrecognized at first glance as the result of a trauma that occurs when Kevin commits his massacres, is in fact a fundamental, non-contingent trajectory of Gnostic revelation, designed to teach Eva the validity of Kevin's antisociality. The film displays all the crucial characteristics of Gnostic myth for Taubes: it depicts an inward turn that detemporalizes myth, recasting it as the self-revelation of the social world as worthy of the most virulent disgust.

I offer this grim reading of the film because it casts ambivalent light on the aesthetic-industrial practice of art house cinema as I discussed it in the first section of this essay. Taubes means his elaboration of Gnostic thought to cast light on how Gnosticism persists in modernity. Generally, attempts to use Gnosticism to address modern texts have addressed artifacts of high culture. Taubes himself links Gnosticism to surrealism (Taubes 2010, p. 101). Other critics have turned to Gnostic ideas to elucidate the works of Joseph Conrad (Henricksen 1978) and Thomas Pynchon (Eddins 1990), and Harold Bloom has argued for Gnosticism as a fundamental heuristic for understanding literary history as a whole (Bloom 1979). The tendency to turn the diagnostic powers of Gnosticism toward high culture, and especially toward modernist artworks, is a reflection and extension of modernism's use of esotericism to shield itself from its own commodity-status. Art house films make similar moves, though in vastly less sophisticated ways. Too much imbrication in the grubby reality of money would diminish the market value of art house films, which present themselves as elevated above mere commodity status by their aesthetic, political, or psychological insights. On the other hand, these very 'insights,' the material of psychosocial realism, impose a coherence on the world that Gnosticism resolutely denies in its understanding that corporeal life is itself a traumatic experience in the strongest sense—an experience of absolute and unbridgeable displacement. The complex narrative structure of *We Need to Talk about Kevin* is an instance of the ambivalent and incomplete turn toward the esoteric that characterizes the industry's uneasy stance on its own production of commodities. The difference between *Kevin*'s narrative and similar modernist gestures in other films is that this film's effort to evade or obscure its own degraded commodity-status presents itself as a revelation of universal degradation. *Kevin* exposes the tension between the aesthetic of realism and the logic

Humanities **2017**, *6*, 90

of trauma. To treat a traumatic event like Kevin's massacre as either a psychological or sociological symptom (the outcome of a culture that glorifies violence or of a woman's resentment of reproductive patriarchy, for example) amounts to taming trauma in the service of rational coherence. The aesthetic of rational explanation that poses as realism in much contemporary American culture stands at odds with the disruption and incoherence that trauma invokes. In the disruptive relationship between the aesthetic-industrial environment in which it participates and its Gnostic content, *Kevin* serves to circle a contradiction in art house film marketing, which seeks to assure audiences of their own superiority to the commodity-world by offering up the 'realness' of that world in the form of psychosocial coherence. I have called attention to Cathy Caruth's understanding of trauma as a failure of knowledge. In her analysis of Freud's *Moses and Monotheism*, Caruth proposes history as a knowledge that stands in the place of the inaccessible knowledge of trauma. The post-structuralist critique of reference, she writes, "is aimed not at eliminating history but at resituating it in our understanding, that is, precisely at permitting *history* to arise where *immediate understanding* may not" (Caruth 1996, p. 11). My account of art house film marketing seeks to find the history that this film's narrative cannot name. What emerges in *Kevin*'s gnostic narrative is a mirror-image of its own status as a commodity that must uphold one Manichean vision of the world (rooted in matters of taste and distinction) by denying another (the melodrama of genre narrative). The world-hating of *We Need to Talk about Kevin* is, in the final analysis, a studied blindness to the marketplace to which films like this nonetheless assiduously address themselves.

Conflicts of Interest: The author declares no conflict of interest.

References

Another Earth. 2011. Directed by Mike Cahill. Los Angeles: Fox Searchlight.

Arendt, Paul. 2006. Ramsay Needs to Shoot a Film About Kevin. *The Guardian*. June 6. Available online: https://www.theguardian.com/film/2006/jun/06/1 (accessed on 11 August 2017).

Bloom, Harold. 1979. Lying Against Time: Gnosis, Poetry, Criticism. *Oxford Literary Review* 3: 4–15.

Box Office Mojo. 2017. Available online: http://www.boxofficemojo.com/studio/chart/?studio= oscilloscopepictures.htm (accessed on 11 August 2017).

Brody, Richard. 2012. We Need to Talk About Kevin. *The New Yorker*. Available online: http://www.newyorker. com/goings-on-about-town/movies/we-need-to-talk-about-kevin-2 (accessed on 11 August 2017).

Caruth, Cathy. 1996. *Unclaimed Experience: Trauma, Narrative, and History*. Baltimore: Johns Hopkins University Press.

Desilets, Sean. 2017. *Hermeneutic Humility and the Political Theology of Cinema: Blind Paul*. New York: Routledge.

Eddins, Dwight. 1990. *The Gnostic Pynchon*. Bloomington: Indiana University Press.

Freud, Sigmund. 1961. *Beyond the Pleasure Principle*. Translated by James Strachey. New York: Norton.

Gold, Joshua Robert. 2006. Jacob Taubes: "Apocalypse from Below". *Telos* 134: 140–56.

Henricksen, Bruce. 1978. 'Heart of Darkness' and the Gnostic Myth. *Mosaic: An Interdisciplinary Critical Journal* 11: 35–44.

Hollywood News. 2010. "We Need to Talk About Kevin" Starts Filming This Week. *Hollywood News*. April 23. Available online: http://www.hollywoodnews.com/2010/04/23/we-need-to-talk-about-kevin-starts-filming-this-week/ (accessed on 11 August 2017).

King, Geoff. 2005. *American Independent Cinema*. Indiana: Indiana University Press.

La historia oficial/The Official Story. 1985. Directed by Luis Puenzo. Washington: Koch-Lorber.

La mujer sin Cabeza/The Headless Woman. 2008. Directed by Lucrecia Martel. Culver City: Strand Releasing.

Martha Marcy May Marlene. 2011. Directed by Sean Durkin. Los Angeles: Fox Searchlight.

Newman, Michael Z. 2009. Indie Culture: In Pursuit of the Authentic Autonomous Alternative. *Cinema Journal* 48: 16–34. [CrossRef]

O Que E Isso, Companheiro?/Four Days in September. 1997. Directed by Bruno Barretos. Santa Monica: Miramax.

O'Regan, Cyril. 2001. *Gnostic Return in Modernity*. New York: SUNY Press.

Rudolph, Kurt. 1987. *Gnosis: The Nature and History of Gnosticism*. Translated by Robert McLachlan Wilson. San Francisco: Harper San Francisco.

Sexton, Jamie. 2012. US "Indie-Horror": Critical Reception, Genre Construction, and Suspect Hybridity. *Cinema Journal* 51: 67–86. [CrossRef]

Shriver, Lionel. 2003. *We Need to Talk about Kevin*. New York: Harper Perennial.

Take Shelter. 2011. Directed by Jeff Nichols. New York: Sony Pictures Classics.

Taubes, Jacob. 2010. *From Cult to Culture: Fragments Toward a Critique of Historical Reason*. Edited by Charlotte Elisheva Fonrobert and Amir Engel. Stanford: Stanford University Press.

The Numbers. 2017. The Numbers: Where Data and the Movie Business Meet. Available online: http://www.the-numbers.com/movies/production-company/Artina-Films and http://www.the-numbers.com/movie/We-need-to-Talk-About-Kevin#tab=summary (accessed on 11 August 2017).

The Sound of My Voice. 2011. Directed by Zal Batmanglij. Los Angeles: Fox Searchlight.

Thomson, David. 2012. Thomson on Film: A Movie About a School Shooting That Ignores the Shooter. *The New Republic*. March 8. Available online: https://newrepublic.com/article/101388/we-need-to-talk-about-kevin-swinton-ramsay-shriver (accessed on 11 August 2017).

Thornham, Sue. 2013. 'A Hatred So Intense . . . ' *We Need to Talk about Kevin*, Postfeminism and Women's Cinema. *Sequence: Serial Studies in Media, Film and Music* 2: 3–38.

Tzioumakis, Yannis. 2012. *Hollywood's Indies: Classics Divisions, Specialty Labels and the Independent Cinema*. Edinburgh: Edinberg University Press.

We Need to Talk About Kevin. 2011. Directed by Lynne Ramsay. Brooklyn: Oscilloscope Pictures.

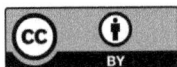

humanities

MDPI

Article

Triangulating Trauma: Constellations of Memory, Representation, and Distortion in Elie Wiesel, Wolfgang Borchert, and W.G. Sebald

William Mahan

German, Davis campus, University of California, Davis, CA 95616, USA; wmmahan@ucdavis.edu

Received: 16 October 2017; Accepted: 19 November 2017; Published: 24 November 2017

Abstract: Even today, trauma theory remains indebted to Sigmund Freud's notion of belatedness: a traumatic event is not fully experienced at the time of occurrence, due to its suddenness and the lack of preparedness on the part of the human subject. In *Traumatic Realism* (2000), Michael Rothberg invokes the Benjaminian notion of the constellation of representation to address the shortcomings of any singular mode of trauma portrayal. Rothberg likens the realist, modernist, and postmodernist literary modes to the points of view of the survivor, the bystander, and the latecomer, respectively. I combine Rothberg's typology with insights from trauma theory to analyze Elie Wiesel's *Night*, Wolfgang Borchert's *The Man Outside*, and W.G. Sebald's *The Emigrants*—three texts that represent Rothberg's literary modes while at the same time problematizing genre. Dori Laub argues that distorted memory and untold stories are endemic to Holocaust representation. W.G. Sebald inscribes this distortion into his narratives, calling attention to but also repeating its effects. I argue that a perspective beginning with (but not limited to) a combined reading of these three texts yields a more complete understanding of trauma and the Holocaust than can be offered by any singular genre—even archives of documented testimonies, which, despite their necessary role, are unavoidably fraught with a problematics of memory itself.

Keywords: Holocaust; representation; postmodernism; collective memory; repression; hypermnesia; testimony; ghosts; realism

---

1. Introduction

As the number of living Holocaust survivors diminishes, society's contact with this trauma becomes increasingly vicarious and necessitates an invigorated engagement in order to preserve its experiential, in addition to its historical, memory. This essay investigates the benefits of an inter-generic approach to the literary representation of trauma, considering the cases of Elie Wiesel's memoir *Night* (*La Nuit* 1958), Wolfgang Borchert's radio play/drama *The Man Outside* (*Draußen vor der Tür* 1947), and the four narratives comprising W.G. Sebald's *The Emigrants* (*Die Ausgewanderten* 1992) as, respectively, testimonial, modernist, and postmodernist voices. I argue that the first two of these modes convey 'post-trauma' effectively, and that postmodernism adds the 'post-post-trauma' perspective to this typology—inherently both advantageous and difficult in its point of view regarding trauma, highlighting its own deficiencies as well as those of documentary/(anti)realist testimony and of modernism. These texts by no means form a complete picture of the typology of trauma representation, in which each source contributes to what might be visualized as a constellation. While on the one hand I argue that they represent the modes described by Michael Rothberg, on the other hand each of these texts complicates genre and extends the boundaries of the constellation of Holocaust representation. Furthermore, a reading of these three texts alongside one another points out the inherent difficulties and disfigurements within each text's approach to trauma, illustrating the merits of comparative and complementary examination. Each of the three texts approaches trauma as memory from a different point of view: autobiographical realism can be seen as the memory of a victim, modernism as that of a witness (often a victim of vicarious trauma), and postmodernism as the next-generation's engagement with (post-)memory.

In *Family Frames: Photography, Narrative, and Postmemory*, Marianne Hirsch recalls a certain picture of a woman named Frieda, wherein, at face level, there is "nothing . . . that indicates its connection to the Holocaust" (Hirsch 1997, p. 19). Yet in the proper context, this picture functions as a "ghostly revenant" (Hirsch 1997, p. 20) not only in the sense that all photographs achieve a return of the past, but also in its connection to the trauma of the Holocaust. This is the primary operative mode of both the images and the text of Sebald's *The Emigrants*: the narratives approach trauma through contextualization rather than through content alone. If Wiesel's *Night* is to find its parallel in images of mass graves, discussed by Hirsch, then *The Emigrants* can be read alongside the picture of the woman Frieda, along with other family photographs of Holocaust victims—the difference is in "the work of reading that they require" (Hirsch 1997, p. 20). This is not to say, however, that Sebald's contextually-dependent text is superior in Holocaust representation to Wiesel's autobiographical depiction, which presents Auschwitz in the immediacy of realism, although it arguably exceeds Wiesel's narrative in complexity. According to Hirsch, "we respond with a similar sense of disbelief" (Hirsch 1997, p. 21) to both generic forms, and thus I argue that a combined reading of trauma influenced by realist, modernist, and postmodernist materials allows one to locate more accurately the phenomenological and ontological consistency of traumatic memory. When read in the context of Wiesel's earlier memoir written in Yiddish, *Un di Velt hot geshvign* (1956), Wiesel's *Night*, written ten years after the fact, takes on new significations that further add to the constellation of representation. To the photographic perspectives offered by Wiesel and Sebald, Borchert's *The Man Outside* adds the sensation of horror experienced not only during the nightmare itself, or in remembering it, but, as Cathy Caruth puts it, "what happens upon waking up" (Caruth 1996, p. 64)—namely, waking consciousness as the reliving of trauma, emphasizing trauma as a break in the mind's experience of time (Caruth 1996, p. 61). Borchert's protagonist Beckmann is thus condemned to walk the earth as a kind of ghost, forced to view life through the metaphor of his wartime respirator glasses.[1]

Central to Caruth's theoretical perspective of trauma is Freud's notion of *Nachträglichkeit* (belatedness), referring to the phenomenon in which memory returns to haunt the victim of a trauma. The return takes place because the violence was not fully understood or known at the time of the traumatic event (Caruth 1996, p. 6). Trauma thus becomes the ongoing experience of having survived death (Caruth 1996, p. 7). Wiesel brings this death back to "life" once again, the *Nachträglichkeit* or delayed onset of his trauma positioned as an offering to the reader of *Night*, whereas Borchert's reader approaches trauma through Beckmann's experience of *Nachträglichkeit* after the fact. In *The Emigrants*, Sebald's task among others is to convey the_burden of *Nachträglichkeit* from one generation to the next. These levels of belatedness find accompaniment also in the level of witnessing. Elie Wiesel represents the first tier of witnessing in Laub's (1995) typology of testimony—namely, *oneself* as a witness. In Michael Rothberg's terms, the self as witness constitutes the point of view of the survivor who attempts to document the undocumentable (Rothberg 2000, p. 13). Borchert's character Beckmann (to an extent) represents the point of view of the bystander, "who feels impelled to bear an impossible witness to the extreme from a place of relative safety," and Sebald's narrator(s) in *The Emigrants* represent(s) the latecomer, or the "representative of the 'postmemory' generation, who, like [Art] Spiegelman, inherits the detritus of the twentieth century" (Rothberg 2000, p. 13). In *Family Frames* (1997), Marianne Hirsch defines postmemory as "the experience of those who grow up dominated by narratives that preceded their birth, whose own belated stories are evacuated by the stories of the previous generation shaped by traumatic events that can be neither understood nor recreated,"

---

[1] One finds a parallel in other Borchert texts in which characters carry other wartime leftovers, such as a kitchen clock in "Die Küchenuhr" ("The Kitchen Clock").

distinguished from original memory by "generational distance" and from history by "deep personal connection" (Hirsch 1997, p. 22). According to Rothberg, these three categories of witness form a constellation that more holistically represents an era of extreme violence and that roughly fits the literary personae of the realist, the modernist, and the postmodernist.[2]

On a microcosmic level, Rothberg identifies all three of these forms as components within a given text's representation of history. The text's realist component thus attempts to document the world; its "modernist" dimension "questions its ability to document history transparently"; and its "postmodern" component "responds to the economic and political conditions of its emergence and public circulation" (Rothberg 2000, p. 9). Rothberg here anticipates an "overlapping of representational modes" (p. 10) in Holocaust studies, advocating for the importance of this overlap. According to Rothberg, one thus avoids the risk of an ahistorical representation of culture that also grasps "historical particularity" (p. 10). He cites Walter Benjamin's "Theses on the Philosophy of History," in which Benjamin conceives of a constellation that links the present to the past. I now begin to connect the points in an interpretive constellation for the representation of Holocaust trauma in Wiesel's, Borchert's, and Sebald's texts.

2. Wiesel: Survivor in the Night

Elie Wiesel's claim that Auschwitz can neither be explained nor visualized, especially in conjunction with Adorno's maxim that writing poetry after Auschwitz is barbaric,[3] problematizes his testimony in *Night*, which attempts to offer an objective, realist account from a survivor's perspective. Although Rothberg takes this claim of Wiesel's—that the Holocaust "transcends history"—as evidence for Wiesel's "antirealist tendency" (Rothberg 2000, p. 5), antirealism in this sense is dependent upon the context of Rothberg's own classification of realists as those who convey the "banality of evil",[4] whereas the antirealists forge "an unbridgeable rupture between the ordinary and the extraordinary" (p. 4). Irrespective of the distance between ordinary events and the uniqueness of the Holocaust, Wiesel's *Night* constitutes realism in the traditional sense, because it attempts to convey his everyday life as it was experienced authentically in Auschwitz. As Rothberg contends, the realist "aims at the mimesis of a certain spatial world," but is "caught in a traumatic temporality" (p. 13). This temporality, for Wiesel personally, creates a belated moral obligation: "to try to prevent the enemy from enjoying one last victory by allowing his crimes to be erased from human memory" (Wiesel [1956] 2006, p. xiii). Despite Wiesel's self-abnegating claim,[5] then, one is able nonetheless to visualize Auschwitz through a reading of *Night*. One thus reaches in Rothberg's typology the category of traumatic realism, which, he argues, mediates between realist and antirealist tendencies and the tensions between the ordinary and the extreme (Rothberg 2000, p. 6). Rothberg's "rethinking of realism" as it applies to Wiesel's *Night* makes apparent the usefulness of accompaniment by modernist and postmodernist texts, each in their own way to be understood as "persistent responses to the demands of history" (Rothberg 2000, p. 9).

In *Night*, Wiesel describes his first day in Auschwitz and the trauma of seeing the bodies of babies being dumped into a burning mass grave: "I pinched myself: Was I alive? Was I awake? How was it possible that men, women, and children were being burned and that the world kept silent? No. All this could not be real. A nightmare perhaps … Soon I would wake up with a start, my heart pounding, and find that I was back in the room of my childhood, with my books…" (Wiesel [1956] 2006, p. 32). Joshua Hirsch sees this moment of trauma for Wiesel as "the moment of finally seeing the unthinkable"

---

[2] Cf. the typology I describe on p. 2.

[3] Theodor Adorno, *Kulturkritik und Gesellschaft* [*Cultural Criticism and Society*] (1951): "Kulturkritik findet sich der letzten Stufe der Dialektik von Kultur und Barbarei gegenüber: nach Auschwitz ein Gedicht zu schreiben, ist barbarisch, und das frißt auch die Erkenntnis an, die ausspricht, warum es unmöglich ward, heute Gedichte zu schreiben" ['Cultural criticism finds itself faced with the final stages of the dialectic of civilization and barbarism. To write poetry after Auschwitz is barbaric. And this corrodes even the knowledge of why it has become impossible to write poetry today' (*Prisms*, p. 34)].

[4] Cf. Hannah Arendt, *Eichmann in Jerusalem* (1963).

[5] His claim that Auschwitz cannot be explained or visualized, cited in Rothberg (2000, p. 13).

and also as an instance of Freud's concept of *Schreck*,[6] which Hirsch translates as "fright," although one might also translate it as terror (Hirsch 2004, pp. 95–96). Wiesel conveys his *Schreck* to the reader of *Night* in the form of traumatic realism, which emphasizes his role as a survivor in the typology of witnesses. His survivor identity also betrays his connection to the present, which occasionally erupts into and interrupts the diegesis of *Night*: "Many years later, in Paris, I sat in the Metro, reading my newspaper. Across the aisle, a beautiful woman with dark hair and dreamy eyes. I had seen those eyes before" (Wiesel [1956] 2006, p. 46). In this episode, as in others, Wiesel achieves narration of the present through its connection to a specific memory from the past: "Years later, I witnessed a similar spectacle in Aden" (Wiesel [1956] 2006, p. 100). To preserve his memory "against his enemy," Wiesel is also unable to erase it from his own life (in the metro station, for example), such that it invades his present-day, narrating self, conjuring Freud's notion of the repetition compulsion.[7] In this way, Wiesel's trauma is not only *nachträglich* for his reader, but as the unanticipated narrative interruptions reveal, also belated for Wiesel himself.

Significantly, Wiesel originally published his memoirs in Yiddish, ten years before the publication of *Night* in French, as discussed for example by Naomi Seidman and Jan Schwarz.[8] Seidman's (1996) article illustrates one way in which one can approach the anti-realist components of *Night*, though on the whole the work still strives to depict a "realist" narrative (as Rothberg indicates, literary texts have various categorical moments both in agreement with and against their general generic flow). The key differences between *Night* and *Un di Velt hot geshvign* laid out by Seidman indeed show a shift in narrative voice concerned with speaking to a different audience. Whereas the earlier text was only one of many in a Yiddish anthology for Jewish readers, *Night* stands on its own and is for a French, European and perhaps global audience. Looking towards Dori Laub's argument, one might venture to claim that Wiesel's desire to be heard was not, and could not be satisfied by *Un di Velt hot geshvign* due to the limitations of his audience. As Laub writes, the "imperative to tell and to be heard can become itself an all-consuming life task. Yet no amount of telling seems ever to do justice to this inner compulsion. There are never enough words or the right words, there is never enough time or the right time, and never enough listening or the right listening to articulate the story that cannot be fully captured in *thought, memory, and speech*" (p. 78). As Seidman describes, *Night* is about one third of the length of the earlier manuscript, but the true difference is in the details, for example Wiesel's desire for Jewish revenge which becomes more suppressed or dismissed by *Night* (p. 5). *Un di Velt hot geshvign* is a more "realist" text in the immediacy of its depiction; still, the matured, distanced perspective of *Night*, especially with the help of the earlier text to aid in memory, offers another "realist," albeit less autobiographically accurate (and confessional) depiction of events (with more fictional license taken). The temporally distanced narrative produced by *Night*, especially in conjunction with the earlier version, instigates a problematics of memory and of (realist) memoir genre, in turn further informing readers' perception of the constellation of Holocaust portrayal.

Theodor Adorno's aforementioned assertion about the impossibility of writing poetry after Auschwitz has frequently been invoked in relation to the limits of Holocaust representation. As Marianne Hirsch points out, one of the consequences of Adorno's assertion has been "the effort to distinguish between the documentary and the aesthetic" (Hirsch 1997, p. 23). Wiesel's retrospective lens raises concern about the divide between documentary factuality and aestheticization within the memory process, especially concerning one's memory (or repression) of trauma. Precisely because Wiesel's autobiographical representation of Auschwitz situates itself as a factual account, the traditional questions about Holocaust writing surface of their own accord: Wiesel's account problematizes "truth and fact, reference and representation, realism and modernism, history and fiction, ethics and politics" (Hirsch 1997, p. 23). Nonetheless, for Marianne Hirsch and her notion of postmemory, Sebald's fictional,

---

[6] See Freud, *Beyond the Pleasure Principle* (1920).
[7] Cf. Freud, *Moses and Monotheism* (1939).
[8] See Schwarz (2007).

photograph-enhanced narratives engage with memory on a level (temporally and generationally) beyond Wiesel's testimony. Joshua Hirsch considers Wiesel's *Night* to belong to a "discourse of trauma" (Hirsch 2004, p. 101). Such discourses of trauma occur for "a society which has suffered a massive blow" and in the period of time "after the initial encounter with a traumatizing historical event but before its ultimate assimilation" (Hirsch 2004, p. 100). The massive blow for the society of Wiesel's trauma discourse is the Holocaust; the image he attempts to convey to the reader is that of the unthinkable. When one encounters such discourse, one comes to understand, according to Hirsch, a "failure of representation" (Hirsch 2004, p. 101). Thus originates a "second phase" in the discourse of trauma in which imagination attempts to measure up to actual experience, "defined less by a particular image content than by the attempt to discover a form for presenting that content which mimics some aspects of PTSD itself" (Hirsch 2004, p. 101). Here, one approaches the works of Borchert and Sebald.

3. Borchert: The Bystander Outside

As a theatrical play, Borchert's *The Man Outside* belongs to a literary form that is traditionally thought of as closer to literary mimesis, or mimicking, of life (than a fictional narrative which tells, rather than shows). This form of mimesis also approximates PTSD in a way that narrative perhaps cannot. Originally a radio play, *The Man Outside* further complicates the notion of genre, declaring itself in its theatrical script a play "which no theatre will produce and no public will want to see" (Borchert [1947] 1971, p. vi). Furthermore, Borchert's writing of the play occurred in temporal immediacy to the war, and the devastation and rubble is transcribed onto the page while it is still fresh (without any sort of belated editing, such as Wiesel's rewriting of his Yiddish memoirs into *Night* for an alternative readership). For Rothberg, the modernist "confronts a particular form of progressive time consciousness, but finds his attempt to establish a before and after frustrated as he is pulled back again and again toward the site of a genocidal crime" (Rothberg 2000, p. 13). Within the diegesis of *The Man Outside*, it is indeed difficult to imagine progress or moving forward, a time "after" the trauma experience. Borchert's protagonist Beckmann's displacement of time consciousness is represented in the metaphor of his respirator glasses.[9] His nightmares as well as his life-as-nightmare embody Ruth Leys's description of the "traumatic nightmare as unclaimed experience" (Leys 2000, p. 272). Although a survivor of Stalingrad like Borchert himself, Beckmann assumes after the war the role of bystander—specifically because those around him refuse to "hear" his testimony. In his transition from survivor to bystander, Beckmann calls attention to the function of seeing. As Dori Laub indicates, the silence resulting from failure to bear witness amounts to a sort of self-imprisonment based on lack. It is appropriate that Borchert begins *The Man Outside* with a prologue scene featuring a dialogue between an old man (God) and Death (the new God) in which the old man lacks a purpose.

Whereas *Night* features occasional intrusions of the present into the past, *The Man Outside* can be characterized as an intrusion of the past into the present, which is also how Joshua Hirsch sees the black and white elements of the Holocaust documentary film *Night and Fog* (Hirsch 2004, p. 117). He likens them to "hypermnesic or hallucinatory episodes; we see too much" (Hirsch 2004, pp. 116–17). Although the film explores the Holocaust in the realm of concentration camps' perpetrators and victims directly, and thus serves as yet another medium that ought to be combined with the texts considered in this essay, an examination of *The Man Outside* offers a more vicarious, neutral experience of a (traumatized) bystander—a German removed from, but privy to the concentration camp experience who experiences horrors of his own on the eastern front. As a bystander and returning soldier, Beckmann attends to Germany's destitute state after the war (and the citizens' ability to come to terms with their war memories), offering the play's listener, viewer, or reader a vision into the experience

---

[9]   To reference another theatrical problematization of time consciousness, Shakespeare's Hamlet constitutes the classic representation of disjointedness of time. In *Specters of Marx*, Jacques Derrida (2006) selects Hamlet as the archetype of his "hauntology," condensed into the claim "The time is out of joint."

through his hypermnesia. This in turn resembles the past's hold on Beckmann, as in his repeating nightmare. Beckmann's is the "troubled gaze of the traumatized witness" (Hirsch 2004, p. 118), representing a post-traumatic consciousness.

Cathy Caruth, in a conversation with Judith Herman, asks about her so-called dialectic of trauma, described as "the simultaneous presence of knowing and not knowing, of intrusive and constrictive symptoms, in traumatic experience, as well as in the social context surrounding trauma and the study of trauma" (Caruth 2014, p. 144). Borchert exposes this dialectic in *The Man Outside*, where Beckmann's "knowing" of his past trauma constricts him when other figures in the play refuse to share in his knowledge. Beckmann is configured as the intruder, a representative of the bodies that float along in the Elbe when society wishes they were hidden beneath the earth. As such, Beckmann manifests the conflict outlined in Herman's "Crime and Memory" referenced in Caruth, namely, "individual disturbances of memory, the amnesias and hypermnesias of traumatized people" (Caruth 2014, p. 144). In this scenario the therapy's success depends on the subject's ability to come to terms with the truth and tell it to an audience, and Beckmann's attempts at telling are denied by refusals to hear. Beckmann is ironically refused amnesia, suffering the yet-worse hypermnesia evidenced by his nightmares and hallucinatory conversations with the "Other". This hypermnesic focus on the past distorts his vision of the present as well as other characters' perceptions of him and willingness to hear him out. As the girl who rescues him from the bank of the Elbe tells him, "Without the glasses you look quite different at once" (Borchert [1947] 1971, p. 92), attributing his discomforting appearance to them. Beckmann responds, "Everything's just a blur to me now. Cough them up. I can't see a thing" (p. 92). As a result of his trauma, which he must witness alone, time is a blur to Beckmann—both the present and the past, because of its imposition into the present. "With the glasses you look like a ghost," the girl tells him, to which he answers: "Perhaps I am a ghost. Yesterday's ghost that no one wants to see today. A ghost from the war, temporarily repaired for peace" (pp. 92–93). Beckmann's self-perceived temporary repair can be understood as a reflection of his sense of duty to bear witness and tell what he has seen.

The play's original title, *Draußen vor der Tür*, can be translated as "Outside, in Front of the Door". Those who find themselves "outside" are "old people who can't adapt themselves to new conditions" (Borchert [1947] 1971, p. 123). As Beckmann laments, "We're all outside. Even God's outside, and no one opens a door to him now. Only death, at the last only death has a door for us" (Borchert [1947] 1971, p. 123). Beckmann's state of being outside the door is ironically exacerbated by the Elbe's refusing his death, as well as by the voice of the Other, who plagues him with an encouraging drive to continue forward but ultimately abandons him when Beckmann puts him to the test of his reasoning. The Other reminds Beckmann of his perpetual state of dreaming, when Beckmann confronts the Colonel with the number of deaths for which he is responsible: "Two thousand and eleven plus Beckmann makes two thousand and twelve. Two thousand and twelve nocturnal ghosts! Brr!" (p. 126). Beckmann's inability to see the present as well as the refusal of others to hear him mark the play with a denial of the senses. In the play's "Prologue," a man arrives in Germany. One reads, "He's been away for a long time, this man. A very long time. Perhaps too long. And he returns quite different from what he was when he went away" (p. 82). It is not stated whether this man is Beckmann or another, allegorical returning soldier, but the effect is the same: the "return," although spatial, does not achieve an ontological domain, and the soldiers "remain" at war, to the extent that their memories of the war continue to traumatize them. As the preface continues, one reads that this man watches a film about another returning soldier, and, as in Wiesel's *Night*, "has to pinch his arm several times during the performance, for he doesn't know whether he's waking or sleeping" (p. 82). In *The Man Outside*, Borchert blurs the distinction between dream and reality to depict trauma as a waking nightmare. For Beckmann, the present day is blurred if he removes his glasses, but he himself is obscured and rendered ghostly to others by these same lenses. Beckmann represents a traumatized nation that is forced also to come to terms with the traumas of the Holocaust for which it is itself the perpetrator, and he suffers from the blindness that can result from such trauma.

4. Sebald: The Latecomer in the (British) Fog

Having examined the means by which realism and modernism (refuse to) represent trauma, be it the Holocaust or the battles of the Second World War, I now turn to W.G. Sebald's *The Emigrants* to consider the crucial perspective that postmodernism's postmemory of trauma adds to the equation. Rothberg writes that the postmodernist "interrogates the reign of the pure image or simulacrum and attempts to negotiate between the demands of memory and the omnipresence of mediation and commodification" (Rothberg 2000, p. 13), and mediation is certainly a key word in paraphrasing the task at hand in Sebald's "novel"—if one elects to characterize the text as such. Consisting of four stand-alone narratives, *The Emigrants* could be seen as four novellas rather than as one novel. Yet all four stories are narrated by a voice that is stylistically indiscernible from the others. The preface to the first narrative within *The Emigrants*, entitled "Dr. Henry Selwyn," reads, "And the last remnants/memory destroys" (Sebald [1992] 1996, p. 1). This sets up the complicated relationship between memory and the ambivalence of erasure and preservation. Whereas Borchert's primary metaphor is Beckmann's respirator glasses, Sebald's is arguably the photograph, especially in the informed, (mis)informing context in which he places the photographs he uses. Osborne characterizes Sebald's engagement with the Holocaust as "oblique" and "indirect" (Osborne 2013, p. 1). So, too, his pictures thematically resemble those family portraits that Marianne Hirsch describes as opposed to those of mass graves—Sebald's images serve as ghostly, indirect references to the Holocaust, for example those of everyday graveyards (as metonymic in relation to mass graves) and a cityscape dominated by chimneys (in relation to concentration camp crematoria). These two images, tellingly, are the first and the last in his narrative (Sebald [1992] 1996, pp. 3, 235).

In responding to "the non-viability of conventional forms of narrative after 1945" (Osborne 2013, p. 1), Sebald seems to agree with Joshua Hirsch's notion of a "failure of representation" (Hirsch 2004, p. 101) of the Holocaust, and could thus be seen as contributing to the second phase of trauma discourse that Hirsch describes. The memories collected by the narrator of each of the stories are often obtained from the removed perspective of other secondary characters who knew the men (Selwyn, Bereyter, Adelwarth, and Ferber). Apparently unconsciously, narrative authority slips back and forth between the narrator and the narrative's interlocutors, a characteristic gesture on Sebald's part, to be observed also in *Austerlitz* (2001). *The Emigrants* can be seen as a text dealing with four separate aftershocks of the same historical rupture. The *Nachträglichkeit* of the men's trauma after the war leads to their deterioration as well as their self-erasures. As a result of Dr. Selwyn's suicide, the narrator of the first episode is also plagued with shock in a manner that can be said to be *nachträglich*: "I had no great difficulty in overcoming the initial shock. But certain things, as I am increasingly becoming aware, have a way of returning unexpectedly, often after a lengthy absence" (Sebald [1992] 1996, p. 23). Sebald constructs his narrative in this manner, with unannounced leitmotifs resurfacing intermittently in the four narratives. One such motif is the freezing and thawing of ice (a metaphor for the preservation and obscurity of memory), and another is the mountain climber Nabokov appearing first in the Selwyn episode and then in "Paul Bereyter". However, another climber makes a perhaps yet more powerful impression on the reader. Naegeli's body thematizes remains, traces, and the return of memory (vis-à-vis the dead), when it is released by the Oberaar glacier seventy-two years after his disappearance. The ice leitmotif is accompanied by one of water, especially shorelines, but also specific places: Lake Geneva surfaces in each of the four narratives as a representation of the tenuous collective memory of Holocaust victims.

As much as Sebald's text appears to be critical of the failure of conventional forms of Holocaust representation, it also emphasizes its own impossibility of success by positing the failure of memory. Nonetheless, Sebald continues to inspire authors such as his contemporary Christoph Ransmayr and the director Christian Petzold, as well as a new generation of present-day artists and authors—all of whom add to the existing constellation of engagement with Holocaust memory. The failure of memory, attached to the metaphor of literal and figurative blindness, is often accompanied by or results from seeing things all too clearly, evoking Joshua Hirsch's linking of amnesia with hypermnesia. Photographs can instigate a literal and emotionally charged return of the past, as the narrator observes in Edwin and Selwyn (Sebald [1992] 1996, pp. 16–17). Ironically, however, this emotion overpowers their sense of time, and the moment of the present invades violently as they stare silently at the picture of themselves for such a long time that the glass in the slide shatters. A dark crack forms across the screen, and in the narrator's memory as well—though later, it vanishes from his mind "almost completely" (Sebald [1992] 1996, p. 17). The problem of first-hand authenticity of witnessing is introduced here, as the narrator concedes; he describes Lasithi as a place that he has himself never seen (p. 18). Lasithi can also be understood as the trauma of the Holocaust, which the second generation simply cannot experience.

History as collective memory also posits the dangers of forgetting, denial, and erasure. The narrator is disappointed that Paul Bereyter's obituary only remarks "that during the Third Reich Paul Bereyter had been prevented from practicing his chosen profession" (Sebald [1992] 1996, p. 27), but gives no further explanation or biographical details, as though history itself slights Bereyter's life story. The reader, however, has the account of the narrator in this instance. That Bereyter dons his old *Wandervogel* windcheater when he commits suicide indicates an imposition of past traumas such that Paul views them not only as formative to his identity, but also as inevitably consuming it. Mme Landau describes her belated reaction to the hints of suicidal tendencies. She tells the narrator, "The disquiet I experienced because of that momentary failure to see what was meant—I now sometimes feel that at that moment I beheld an image of death—lasted only a very short time, and passed over me like the shadow of a bird in flight" (Sebald [1992] 1996, p. 63). The bird's shadow functions similarly to a photograph, described by Hirsch as containing "simultaneous presence of life and death" (Hirsch 1997, p. 19). Sebald's narrator describes the effects of such photographs on him personally: he leafs through the album over and over, returning to it years later. He finds that it seemed then, and indeed it still seems "as if the dead were coming back, or as if we were on the point of joining them" (Sebald [1992] 1996, p. 46). The ghosts of the previous generation thus haunt the narrator through these photographs as well as in his memory.

Paul's eyes worsen, seemingly in connection with the trauma that he witnessed during the *Kristallnacht* as a child, but which has been repressed in his unconscious. After Bereyter's eyes are bandaged following an operation for cataracts, he admits "that he could [now] see things then with the greatest clarity, as one sees them in dreams, things he had not thought he still had within him" (Sebald [1992] 1996, p. 51). The surgeon prescribes looking at leaves to improve his eyesight. However, according to Mme Landau, Paul disregarded the doctor's orders at night, reading works by authors who "had taken their own lives or been close to doing so" as a result of the war (p. 58). Eventually, the condition of Paul's eyes "began to deteriorate," until "all he could see were fragmented or shattered images" (p. 59), recalling the shattered glass slide from the Dr. Selwyn episode.

Sebald begins the Adelwarth episode by calling attention to the failure of memory: "I have barely any recollection of my own of Great-Uncle Adelwarth," the narrator writes (Sebald [1992] 1996, p. 67). Because memory fails, the narrative shifts quickly to other authorities, but when Aunt Theres departs for America, disappears as easily as memory or as arbitrarily as the past—"for ever, as one might say" (Sebald [1992] 1996, p. 69). The narrator, as a result, forgets his own *dreams* of America. Instead, he becomes interested in what appears to have been his great-uncle's desire "to escape the conventional structures of family, home, and community, structures which want to root the individual in a spatial sense, but also in terms of history" (Osborne 2013, p. 105). Aunt Fini seems, to an extent out of her own sadness and trauma, to refuse to participate in the genealogical and epistemological excavating of Adelwarth but passes this task on to the narrator.[10] The diary of Adelwarth's that Aunt Fini gives the narrator is written in a plethora of languages and in poor handwriting, making its decoding a substantial challenge. Aunt Fini's poor eyesight replicates the metaphor of blindness and vision in

---

[10] She offers the narrator a photo of Adelwarth taken while they were in Jerusalem as well as a diary that she claims not to have been able to decipher herself.

connection to memory and recalls Bereyter's condition. Nonetheless, she is able to recall and share, quite vividly, the details of the relationship between Adelwarth and Cosmo Solomon. Cosmo, in turn, experienced episodes in which "he would be so beside himself that he no longer even recognized Ambros. And yet he claimed that he could see clearly, in his own head, what was happening in Europe: the inferno, the dying, the rotting bodies lying in the sun in open fields" (Sebald [1992] 1996, p. 95). The metaphor of vision here is manifested in near-sighted and far-sighted components. According to Aunt Fini, Adelwarth and Cosmo's visit to Egypt "was an attempt to regain the past, an attempt that appears to have failed in every respect" (pp. 96–97).[11] As with the other emigrants, attempts both to regain and to forget the traumatic past ultimately fail for this generation.

The narrator himself becomes a sort of ghost in this episode, travelling to "what was once the most luxurious hotel on the coast of Normandy," which is now "a monumental monstrosity half sunk in the sand" (Sebald [1992] 1996, p. 118). The few other guests at the hotel are also ghosts, "indestructible ladies who come every summer and haunt the immense edifice. They pull the white dustsheets off the furniture for a few weeks and at night, silent on their biers, they lie in the empty midst of it" (p. 118). White dust sheets often signify spaces haunted by memories, usually in private houses, although hotels are frequently haunted domains as well. Tellingly, the narrator is haunted on this night of his stay in the hotel by Cosmo and Ambros in a dream in which he is crossing the Atlantic, though they remain silent. When he tries to approach them, "they dissolved before my very eyes, leaving behind them nothing but the vacant space they occupied" (p. 123). All of the emigrants similarly dissolve from existence, although they have been preserved in narrative and photographic memory.

Of Sebald's characters, Max Ferber (or Aurach in the original German) represents "the most tangible link to the Holocaust" (Osborne 2013, p. 107), having escaped to England although his parents were deported to a camp and murdered. In this sense, Ferber's trauma was the least vicarious of the men belonging to the postwar generation under investigation by the narrating figure. Perhaps even more telling is the fact that W.G. (Winfried Georg) also went by Max Sebald, and personally felt a sense of vicarious trauma in connection to the Holocaust. The narrator seeks Ferber out in Manchester, which he describes as uncannily empty. The woman who lets him into his lodging has a "Lorelei-like air about her" (Sebald [1992] 1996, p. 152), and even on Saturday evening in the city, "there was no sign of life" (p. 155), as though the only residents were ghosts (recalling the Normandy hotel in the Adelwarth episode). Visiting Ferber, the narrator learns that the dust that is a byproduct of his painting "was the true product of his continuing endeavors and the most palpable proof of his failure" (p. 161). Ferber's technique involves "constantly erasing" (p. 162), but in the process also creates the sense of a genealogy of faces left behind in each new one. Creating and rejecting his own history in his art, Ferber seems to become the dust that results: "He felt closer to dust, he said, than to light, air or water" (p. 161). He tells the narrator about a man who absorbed so much silver in his photographic lab career "that he had become a kind of photographic plate" (p. 165), and it seems that Ferber sees his own fate as similar. A memory of a slipped disk and "the crooked position" he was forced to stand in reminds him also of a photograph his father took of him when he had been bent over his writing: "I began to remember, and it was probably those recollections that prompted me to go on to Lake Geneva after eight days, to retrace another old memory that had long been buried and which I had never dared disturb" (p. 172). Though Ferber does not explicitly reveal this second old memory here, we learn over the next twenty or so pages that he is painfully remembering his childhood, in which his family was

---

11 The trip to Egypt is also likely a reference to Ingeborg Bachmann's *Der Fall Franza* (*The Case of Franza*) (1966)—another account of the violent aftershocks of trauma.

deported to Dachau.[12] As a result of this recovery, Ferber comes to an ultimate judgment of Germany as a country.

Ferber tells the narrator that Germany is "frozen in the past, destroyed, a curiously extraterritorial place, inhabited by people whose faces are both lovely and dreadful" (p. 181). Rather than the blindness of forgetting, "he could see it all with painful clarity" (pp. 187–88). Yet the picture we see a few pages later, of a haunted-looking Victorian house, features a girl in front of the house whose face is blurred. And Ferber, too, tells of the barrier that is beginning to coagulate in front of his view of the past as a result of what he sees to be failed collective German memory: "I felt increasingly that the mental impoverishment and lack of memory that marked the Germans, and the efficiency with which they had cleaned everything up, were beginning to affect my head and my nerves" (p. 225). For Ferber, the speed with which Germany moved beyond the Holocaust added to the traumas of his youth, including the deportation of immediate family to Dachau.

5. Conclusions

In many ways, Sebald works with the remnants of the memories that comprise Wiesel's text and haunt Borchert's. The ghosts in *The Emigrants* belong to the realm of postmemory, which Marianne Hirsch describes as "as full and as empty, certainly as constructed, as memory itself" (Hirsch 1997, p. 22). Hirsch's notion of postmemory is indebted to Henri Raczymow's "mémoire trouée," his "memory shot through with holes" (Hirsch 1997, p. 23), and finds its embodiment in the photograph. Hirsch characterizes the connection between photographs and life as "umbilical" (p. 23), a designation which also stages the intergenerational function of photographs. In *The Emigrants* many photographs have vanished, while the remaining ones must be tracked down. Once again, we face the question of whether Sebald's *The Emigrants* is superior to Borchert's *The Man Outside* or Wiesel's *Night*—whether Sebald's indirect approach to (Holocaust) trauma conveys it more accurately. Dominick LaCapra argues that "history is a field of framed hyperbole" (LaCapra 2001, pp. 194–95) and thus one might be inclined to favor Sebald's hyperbolic postmodernism. However, LaCapra also points out that "history faces the problem of both writing about and writing out trauma" (p. 194), and given this pattern of trauma in history, one ultimately turns back towards Benjamin's notion of time (the past and present) as a constellation. As with Marianne Hirsch's emphasis on the role of context for the photograph of the woman Frieda, Sebald's *Emigrants*, too, requires appropriate contextualization. As different expressions of the same collective trauma, the three texts examined contextualize one another, demonstrating the significance of comparing various representations of the Holocaust to understand its experience as completely and preserve its memory as holistically as possible.

Conflicts of Interest: The author declares no conflict of interest.

References

Borchert, Wolfgang. 1971. *The Man Outside*. Translated by David Porter. New York: New Directions. First broadcast and published in 1947.

Caruth, Cathy. 1996. *Unclaimed Experience: Trauma, Narrative, and History*. Baltimore: Johns Hopkins University Press.

Caruth, Cathy. 2014. *Listening to Trauma: Conversations with Leaders in the Theory and Treatment of Catastrophic Experience*. Baltimore: Johns Hopkins University Press.

Derrida, Jacques. 2006. *Specters of Marx: The State of Debt, the Work of Mourning, and the New International*. Translated by Peggy Kamuf. New York: Routledge.

---

12 Ferber then recounts his father taking him up the Jungfraujoch to the largest glacier in Europe, telling the narrator that he recollected these memories on his train journey through Switzerland thirty years after the fact. During this later visit, Ferber recalls, he was led down the mountain in his state of dizziness with a man with a butterfly net (here, Sebald draws inspiration from Walter Benjamin's *Berlin Childhood around 1900*). In this roundabout way, Ferber approaches his childhood traumas, including the deportation of his family to Dachau.

Hirsch, Marianne. 1997. *Family Frames: Photography, Narrative, and Postmemory*. Cambridge: Harvard University Press.

Hirsch, Joshua. 2004. Post-traumatic Cinema and the Holocaust Documentary. In *Trauma and Cinema: Cross Cultural Explorations*. Edited by E. Ann Kaplan and Ban Wang. Hong Kong: Hong Kong University Press, pp. 93–121.

LaCapra, Dominick. 2001. *Writing History, Writing Trauma*. Baltimore: Johns Hopkins University Press.

Laub, Dori. 1995. Truth and Testimony: The Process and the Struggle. In *Trauma: Explorations in Memory*. Edited by Cathy Caruth. Baltimore: Johns Hopkins University Press, pp. 61–75.

Leys, Ruth. 2000. *Trauma: A Genealogy*. Chicago: University of Chicago Press.

Osborne, Dora. 2013. *Traces of Trauma in W.G. Sebald and Christoph Ransmayr*. Leeds: Modern Humanities Research Association.

Rothberg, Michael. 2000. *Traumatic Realism: The Demands of Holocaust Representation*. Minneapolis: University of Minnesota Press.

Schwarz, Jan. 2007. The Original Yiddish Text and the Context of Night. In *Approaches to Teaching Wiesel's Night*. Edited by Alan Rosen. New York: Modern Language Association of America, pp. 52–58.

Sebald, W. G. 1996. *The Emigrants*. Translated by Michael Hulse. New York: New Directions. First published in 1992.

Seidman, Naomi. 1996. Elie Wiesel and the Scandal of Jewish Rage. In *Jewish Social Studies*. Champagne: Illinois University Press, pp. 1–19.

Wiesel, Elie. 2006. *Night*. Translated by Marion Wiesel. New York: Hill and Wang. First published in 1956.

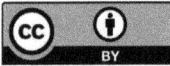

humanities

MDPI

Article

Trauma, Postmemory, and Empathy: The Migrant Crisis and the German Past in Jenny Erpenbeck's *Gehen, ging, gegangen* [*Go, Went, Gone*]

Brangwen Stone

Department of International Studies, Macquarie University, Sydney, NSW 2109, Australia;
brangwen.stone@mq.edu.au

Academic Editor: Gail Finney
Received: 25 September 2017; Accepted: 7 November 2017; Published: 11 November 2017

Abstract: The novel *Gehen, ging, gegangen* [*Go, Went, Gone*] by the celebrated German writer Jenny Erpenbeck was published at the height of the European refugee crisis. The novel tells the tale of Richard, a retired Berlin classics professor, who becomes intrigued by the Oranienplatz refugee protest camp. He initially approaches the refugee crisis as a new research project, methodically searching for secondary literature, composing questionnaires and conducting interviews with asylum seekers, but eventually he begins to develop friendships with some of them. Throughout the novel, Richard, who fled from the approaching Red Army with his mother as a baby and then lived in the German Democratic Republic (GDR) until reunification, notices similarities between the traumatic experiences of the Oranienplatz protesters and the trauma in his personal history, German collective history, and ancient and medieval literature. This article focuses on trauma and empathy in *Gehen, ging, gegangen*, exploring how the parallels drawn between the varied fates of the asylum seekers and the stories of exile and displacement in the literary canon, and German historical experiences of displacement and loss of home, establish points of empathic connection between Richard and the refugees, and attempt to establish the same between the reader and the refugees.

Keywords: trauma; postmemory; empathy; German literature; refugee; Erpenbeck; *Gehen, ging, gegangen*; *Go, Went, Gone*

1. Introduction

The novel *Gehen, ging, gegangen* [*Go, Went, Gone*] by the celebrated German writer Jenny Erpenbeck was published in the late summer of 2015 at the peak of the European refugee crisis, a week before Angela Merkel opened Germany's borders to refugees. It was hailed variously as the *Roman der Stunde* ['novel of the hour'] (Von Sternburg 2015), *Roman der Saison* ['novel of the season'] (Magenau 2015), and *Roman zur politischen Situation* ['novel for the political situation'] (Lühmann 2015) in reviews, although it was based on earlier events. The novel centers on Richard, a widowed Berlin classics professor, who has recently retired. Leading a mundane and somewhat lonely existence, he becomes intrigued by the refugees occupying Oranienplatz (a public square in the central Berlin neighbourhood of Kreuzburg), after first becoming aware of the refugee protests due to a hunger strike on Alexanderplatz. According to a recently published UNHCR report, the number of refugees registered worldwide in 2016 was greater than ever before (UNHCR 2017). Yet, the trauma and anguish experienced by the millions of refugees currently displaced from their homes are not unprecedented. Stories of involuntary displacement have been told since the beginning of time. Narratives of flight and exile are central to a range of canonical texts, including Homer's *Odyssey*, to which Erpenbeck's narrator Richard refers several times, Virgil's *Aeneid*, the *Bible*, the *Qu'ran*, and the modernist novels written by "exiles and émigrés" (Eagleton 1970). The twentieth century saw millions of people forced from their homes as a result of political upheaval on an unprecedented scale, including two world wars, the Cold War, and decolonization. Thus Edward Said declared the twentieth century "the age of the refugee, the displaced person, [and] mass immigration" (Said 2002, p. 159). Equally, the figure of the refugee became one of Giorgio Agamben's key examples to illustrate that "[t]he fundamental categorical pair of Western politics is not that of friend/enemy but that of bare life/political existence, *zoē/bios*, exclusion/inclusion" (Agamben 1998, p. 8).[1] Yet, as Aleida Assmann notes, the phenomenon of forced dislocation has not yet been sufficiently integrated into collective European memory:

> *Die Erfahrung von Flucht, Vertreibung und Migration hat noch keine klare Kontur und Symbolik in der europäischen Erinnerungskultur erhalten. Dafür fehlt vorerst noch ein Narrativ und das liegt wohl nicht zuletzt daran, dass es sich hier um eine im wahrsten Sinne des Wortes 'unendliche Geschichte' handelt, die sich in ganz unterschiedlichen historischen Kontexten wiederholt.*

> The experience of flight, expulsion and migration has no clear contours or symbolism in European memory culture yet. The narrative necessary for this to be the case does not yet exist, not least because it is a "never-ending story" in the truest sense of the word, which repeats itself in very different historical contexts.'[2] (Assmann 2016a).

This article will focus on the role of trauma and empathy in *Gehen, ging, gegangen*, exploring how the parallels drawn between the varied fates of the Oranienplatz asylum seekers and the stories and experiences of exile and displacement in the literary canon, and German history, establish points of empathic connection between Richard and the refugees, and attempt to establish the same between the reader and the refugees.

2. The Occupation of Oranienplatz

The occupation of Oranienplatz on which Erpenbeck based *Gehen, ging, gegangen* began in the autumn of 2012 and lasted for 550 days. The 100–150 protesters, who came from "Sudan, Uganda, Syria, Eritrea, Somalia, Afghanistan and other nations converted [the] square into an urban campsite that served as a loaded space for social and political discussion and negotiation" (Landry 2015, p. 399). The wave of protests that eventually resulted in the protest camp was triggered by the suicide of an Iranian asylum seeker in Würzburg in early 2012, to which protesters reacted with a hunger strike (Wiedemann 2015). By the late summer of 2012, there were tent protests against German refugee policy and the poor conditions in many homes for asylum seekers in most major German cities (Landry 2015, pp. 400–2). In early September, a 28-day march from Würzburg to Berlin followed. On arrival in Berlin, the asylum seekers and their supporters initially set up camp on Pariser Platz next to the Brandenburger Tor, but a move to Oranienplatz was soon negotiated at the invitation of the then mayor of Kreuzberg-Friedrichshain, Franz Schulz of the Green Party (Landry 2015, pp. 402–3). A few months later, as winter began, a number of the refugee activists moved to the nearby abandoned Gerhart-Hauptmann school (Bhimji 2016, p. 9). The occupation of Oranienplatz ended in April 2014, when the protesters were persuaded to move to temporary accommodation with the promise that their applications for asylum would be expedited (Fadaee 2015, p. 735). Some protesters refused to clear the Oranienplatz, and the female Sudanese activist Napuli Langa, whose actions are briefly alluded to by Erpenbeck (Erpenbeck 2015, p. 4), spent five nights in a tree (Wiedemann 2015). A number of protesters continued to occupy part of the Gerhart-Hauptmann school at the time this essay was written (Gehrke 2017). The occupation of Oranienplatz brought the plight of asylum seekers to public attention in Berlin and throughout Germany, and is thought to have been a deciding factor in the lifting of the *Residenzpflicht* (residence duty), which prevented asylum seekers from leaving the state

---

[1] Imogen Tyler warns that the "theoretical turn to the figure of the refugee or asylum seeker within disciplines such as philosophy and cultural studies risks becoming a means of not hearing asylum seekers" (Tyler 2006, p. 199).

[2] All translations in this article are the author's own, unless otherwise noted.

where they registered, and also in the introduction of a new rule allowing asylum seekers the right to work in Germany after a restricted period (Landry 2015, p. 410).[3]

3. The Oranienplatz Protesters in *Gehen, ging, gegangen*

In *Gehen, ging, gegangen*, Richard, a widowed, recently-retired professor who shares the narration of the novel with other characters and an omniscient third-person narrator, is at a loss as to how to fill his days. He initially approaches the refugee crisis as a new research project to replace what retirement has taken away. At first he methodically searches for secondary literature, composes questionnaires, and conducts interviews with asylum seekers, but eventually he begins to develop friendships with some of them. Erpenbeck has stated that the novel is based on similar interviews she herself undertook with the Oranienplatz protesters (Bartels 2015). Throughout the novel, Richard, who fled Silesia from the approaching Red Army with his mother as a baby and then lived in the German Democratic Republic (GDR) until reunification, remembers elements of his own life. He notices similarities between the experiences of the asylum seekers and his personal history, but also parallels with German collective history, ranging from World War II to the subsequent flights, expulsions and deprivations; life under surveillance in the GDR, to the fall of the Berlin Wall and life in the reunified Germany. As an emeritus classics professor, he is also reminded of the narratives of exile and displacement in the ancient literary canon, alluding on numerous occasions to Odysseus and the *Odyssey*, for instance (Erpenbeck 2015, pp. 13, 32–33, 73, 187).

Richard's interest in the Oranienplatz asylum seekers is not triggered until more than a year into the protest, after hearing three pieces of news. First, he hears of a hunger strike on the Alexanderplatz (Erpenbeck 2015, pp. 20, 27), and soon after, in short succession, he learns of the sinking of a boat filled with refugees off the island of Lampedusa, and of the Oranienplatz protests (Erpenbeck 2015, p. 33). He starts researching the countries of origin of the refugees who drowned near Lampedusa (Erpenbeck 2015, pp. 33–34). A few days later he visits Oranienplatz and sees "*[e]ine Landschaft aus Zelten, Bretterbuden und Planen: weiß, blau und grün*" (Erpenbeck 2015, p. 44) ['a landscape of tents, wooden shacks and tarps: white, blue and green' (Erpenbeck 2017, chp. 8)]. He sits down and observes the interactions of the black refugees and their white supporters for two and a half hours without talking to them (Erpenbeck 2015, pp. 44–50). After his visit to Oranienplatz, his research project begins in earnest, "*[d]ie nächsten zwei Wochen verwendet Richard darauf, einige Bücher zum Thema zu lesen und einen Fragenkatalog für die Gespräche, die er mit den Flüchtlingen führen will, zu entwerfen*" (Erpenbeck 2015, p. 51) ['Richard spends the next two weeks reading several books on the subject of the refugees and drawing up a catalog of questions for the conversations he wants to have with them' (Erpenbeck 2017, chp. 9)]. The next time he visits Oranienplatz, he arrives just in time "*um zu sehen, wie auf dem abgesperrten und von Polizei umstellten Platz die letzten Bretter, Planen, Matratzen und Pappen von einem Bagger zusammengeschoben, auf LKWs verladen und fortgeschafft wurden*" (Erpenbeck 2015, p. 54) ['to see the last of the boards, tarps, mattresses, and cardboard signs being shoved into a heap by a bulldozer, loaded onto trucks and carted away' (Erpenbeck 2017, chp. 10)].

4. The Refugees' Stories

It is only now, after the asylum seekers have left the Oranienplatz and have been moved to other housing, that Richard actually speaks to them. Using his painstakingly constructed questionnaire, he interviews them individually, but also gradually forms relationships that go beyond his research project, letting one play his piano, giving another odd jobs around the house, and purchasing a property in Ghana for the family of a third (Erpenbeck 2015, p. 282). Richard delves into the details of

---

[3] As Imogen Tyler and Katarzyna Marciniak note, the paradox of such protests is that although they "are 'acts' against the exclusionary technologies of citizenship, which aim to make visible the violence of citizenship as *regimes of control*," "protestors are compelled to make their demands in the idiom of the regime of citizenship they are contesting" in order to effect material change (Marciniak and Tyler 2013, p. 146).

the refugees' places of origin, their lives, their suffering and the histories of their countries of origin, going back to ancient times. Many of the refugees' stories, as conveyed to Richard, are told in detail, some of them filling whole chapters. The stories uncovered are varied and horrendous: Raschid, for instance, was saved from a shipwreck in which 550 of the 800 asylum seekers on the boat, including his own children, drowned (Erpenbeck 2015, pp. 61–62, 240). This followed fleeing Nigeria as a child when his father was burnt alive in his own car (Erpenbeck 2015, p. 112). Another refugee, whom Richard dubs Apoll, is a Tuareg orphan and former child slave, covered in scars from the beatings of his so-called family (Erpenbeck 2015, pp. 67–68). Many of the protesters recall seeing how their friends and families were slaughtered before they fled. As will gradually become clear towards the end of the novel—or may be clear to those familiar with refugee politics from the beginning—most of the Oranienplatz protesters will not be recognized as refugees despite the persecution they have suffered, due to the vagaries and specificities of both German refugee law and international treaties relating to asylum seekers.

The narratives of the refugees' lives are punctuated by the links Richard makes to other similar experiences in his life, in recent history, and in literature. As the novel progresses and the refugees become his friends and acquaintances, these connections gradually move from references to the ancient and medieval literary canon to allusions that are more contemporary or more personal. The refugees' experiences remind the emeritus professor, of various episodes including his mother's flight from Silesia with him as a baby (Erpenbeck 2015, pp. 25–26); his father's role as a soldier in World War II; and his mother's time as a *Trümmerfrau*[4] (Erpenbeck 2015, pp. 118–19). Ghanaian Awad's mother died in childbirth, which is reminiscent of Blanchefleur dying when Tristan was born, while Awad's flight from the war in Libya, where he later lived with his father, leads Richard to think of both the long history of German wars encapsulated in the children's song "*Maikäfer flieg, mein Vater ist im Krieg*" (Erpenbeck 2015, p. 82) ['Cockchafer Fly! Your father's off at war!' (Erpenbeck 2017, chp. 14)], and of the exile of Goethe's Iphigenia to Tauris (Erpenbeck 2015, pp. 82–83). Later, Apoll's decision to ration his consumption of couscous—consuming only a quarter of a modest plate per day—to ensure that he will not become as helpless as a newborn baby so that he can cope if he is deprived of food and water again, reminds Richard of a TV documentary in which a Jewish girl decides to prepare herself for the Polish camps by wearing light shoes in midwinter before deportation (Erpenbeck 2015, pp. 218–19). Another refugee's explanation that he and his best friend decided to split up and find their own way once they arrived in Europe, thinking "*vielleicht hat wenigstens einer von uns Glück und kann dann später dem anderen helfen*" (Erpenbeck 2015, p. 221) ['one of us might get lucky and then that person could help the other one' (Erpenbeck 2017, chp. 38)], leads Richard to a more general association of the fate of the refugees' with that of the German people historically: "*[e]s ist noch nicht so lange her […] da war die Geschichte der Auswanderung und der Suche nach Glück eine deutsche Geschichte*" (Erpenbeck 2015, p. 222) ['Not so long ago […] the story of going abroad to find one's fortune was a German one' (Erpenbeck 2017, chp. 38)].

Spiegel reviewer Dana Buchzik rejected these allusions, emphasizing the incommensurability of flight:

> *Auch Blanscheflur starb bei Tristans Geburt, konstatiert der emeritierte Professor, als ein verwaister Flüchtling ihm seine Geschichte erzählt. Auch Mozarts Tamino wurde geprüft und davon abgehalten, weiterzugehen, sinniert Richard, auch Goethes Iphigenie war letztlich Emigrantin auf Tauris—auf den Gedanken, dass zwischen Emigration und Flucht ein Unterschied bestehen könnte, kommt Erpenbecks Protagonist nicht.*[5]

---

[4] *Trümmerfrauen*—literally 'rubble women'—were women who cleared the rubble from bombed German cities after World War II.

[5] Stefan Hermes supports her interpretation, focusing on the connections Richard makes between the traumatic experiences of the asylum seekers and those of characters in the European literary canon, and deeming them "*denkbar unangemessen, ja zum Teil beinahe lächerlich*" ['conceivably inappropriate, and in some instances even ludicrous'] (Hermes 2016). Both Buchzik

'The emeritus professor notes that Blanchefleur also died during Tristan's birth, when an orphaned refugee tells him his story. Mozart's Tamino was also put to the test, and hindered from venturing further, Richard ruminates, Goethe's Iphigenia was also an emigrant on the peninsula of Tauris—it does not occur to Erpenbeck's protagonist that there could be a difference between emigration and flight.' (Buchzik 2015).

This critique suggests that Erpenbeck's emphasis on the universality of the suffering the refugees have experienced, and are experiencing, flattens difference. It is undeniable that Erpenbeck emphasizes commonalities, yet the stories of the refugees told in *Gehen, ging, gegangen* are also stories of the particular, featuring the specific experiences of asylum seekers from a diverse range of cultural and religious backgrounds and going beyond the mass concept of the 'refugee', which as Said notes, suggests "large herds of innocent and bewildered people requiring urgent international assistance" (Said 2002, p. 181).

5. Empathy

Instead of eliding difference, Erpenbeck is, it seems, trying to trigger the reader's empathy towards asylum seekers,[6] at a time of increasing concern about Germany's acceptance of refugees and of rising xenophobia.[7] Assmann and Ines Detmers argue in their introduction to their edited volume *Empathy and its Limits* that "empathy is a new topic," pointing out both that it is a recent topic in a number of disciplines, and also that there has been very little interaction between different disciplines' approaches to it (Assmann and Detmers 2016, p. 1). Yet, literature has long been regarded as playing an important role in the development of empathy.[8] Susan Sontag, for instance, argues that the "ability to weep for those who are not us or ours" is exactly what literary narratives can "train" (Sontag 2007, p. 205), while Martha Nussbaum contends that the genre of the novel in particular, "on account of some general features of its structure, generally constructs empathy and compassion in ways highly relevant to citizenship" (Nussbaum 1995, p. 10).

Furthermore, as Stef Craps notes, the concept of empathy "plays a crucial role in much recent work on trauma and witnessing" (Craps 2008, p. 191). Empathy is, for instance, central to Alison Landsberg's theory of 'prosthetic memory', which was first developed in relation to mass media events but which has proven useful in reference to literature too. She defines prosthetic memories as "privately felt public memories that develop after an encounter with a mass cultural representation of the past, when new images and ideas come into contact with a person's own archive of experience" (Landsberg 2004, p. 19). Landsberg argues that "even memories of events that one did not live through can be affectively charged and therefore have the potential to produce empathy and to alter an individual's political commitments" (Landsberg 2015, p. 149). She explains further that "empathy is about developing compassion not for our family or friends or community, but for others—others

---

and Hermes focus on the parallels drawn to the literary canon, not mentioning those drawn to Richard's personal history and German collective history.

[6] Some reviewers commented on this point, Jörg Magenau, for instance wrote: *"Die didaktische Absicht […] ist klar: der anonymen Menge der Flüchtlinge persönliche Gesichter und Geschichten zu verleihen, um so die Empathie zu steigern"* ['The didactic intention […] is clear: to lend the anonymous refugee masses personal faces and stories, and thus to increase empathy'] (Magenau 2015). Friedmar Apel, on the other hand, disagreed: *"Obwohl diese Geschichten sehr bewegend sind, appelliert 'Gehen, ging, gegangen' nicht vordergründig an das Mitleid des Lesers"* ['Although these stories are very moving, "Gehen, ging, gegangen" does not ostensibly appeal to the compassion of the reader'] (Apel 2015).

[7] In a recent telephone survey, 65% of Germans reported that they felt less safe than 2 years ago (Stockrahm 2017); at the same time xenophobic attacks on foreigners have risen (*Die Zeit* 2016), with more than 3500 attacks in 2016 (*Der Spiegel* 2017). Political scientist Robert Vehrkamp makes a clear connection between the arrival of refugees and support for the right-wing populist AfD (Alternative for Germany) party, arguing that the rise in AfD support in 2015 was related to the refugee crisis, and that the fall in their poll numbers in early 2017 was the result of the fact that the refugee crisis was no longer the dominant theme in German politics (Fieber 2017).

[8] As has theatre, which is why Brecht famously used *Verfremdungseffekte* (alienation effects) to avoid awakening empathy in his audience. Jill Bennett relates Dominick LaCapra's notion of empathic unsettlement, discussed below, to Bertolt Brecht's critique of crude empathy (Bennett 2005, p. 10).

who have no relation to us, who resemble us not at all, whose circumstances lie far outside of our own experiences" (Landsberg 2009, p. 223). Dominick LaCapra also makes the link between empathy and the remembrance of traumatic events, emphasizing the importance of empathy for writing about traumatic historical events. He argues that historians (and fiction writers) should approach traumatic historical experiences with "empathic unsettlement," which avoids both the pitfalls of numbing and of "unchecked identification, vicarious experience and surrogate victimage" (LaCapra 2001, p. 40). According to LaCapra, "[e]mpathy in this sense is a form of virtual, not vicarious, experience, related to what Kaja Silverman has termed *heteropathic identification*, in which emotional response comes with respect for the other and the realization that the experience of the other is not one's own" (LaCapra 2001, p. 40; Silverman 1996). Although Buchzik's review of *Gehen, ging, gegangen* suggests that in her opinion Erpenbeck, or at least her narrator Richard, has fallen into the trap of 'unchecked identification' identified by LaCapra, a clear distinction is always made between the experiences of the individual refugees, on the one hand, and Richard and the other Western figures—fictional or otherwise— to whom their experiences are linked, on the other.[9]

Amos Goldberg argues, drawing on Hannah Arendt's work on the refugee and the modern nation state after World War II, that "empathy towards the refugee presents such a great challenge and is so unsettling, since it is directed at the traumatic element within the modern nation state" (Goldberg 2016, p. 71). In this understanding the refugee represents the 'other' of the modern nation state, thus challenging and undermining it. Although theoretical writings on empathy in both literary and trauma theory underline the importance of difference being acknowledged for empathy to be felt (as opposed to sympathy, which is based on similarity), they largely focus on empathy being felt by those in the West towards Western literary figures or historical victims of trauma. Yet most of the asylum seekers arriving in Germany in recent times, such as the group of protesters portrayed in *Gehen, ging, gegangen* who stem from Africa and the Middle East, are not from the West. As Judith Butler notes, those in the West are less likely to feel empathy for non-Westerners, as signified by the way in which the loss of different kinds of lives are treated. Butler argues that while some lives are publically acknowledged and grieved, other lives (for instance AIDS deaths or the large numbers of people dying in Africa) are "unmarkable" and "ungrievable" (Butler 2004, p. 35). Butler contends that the narratives in the Western media "stage the scene and provide the narrative means by which 'the human' in its grievability is established" (Butler 2004, p. 38). Susannah Radstone makes a similar argument in relation to trauma theory, noting that while certain events are labeled traumatic, others "quite patently" are not (Radstone 2007, p. 25). Moreover, she argues, "it is the sufferings of those categorized, in the West as 'other', that tend *not* to be addressed via trauma theory—which becomes in this regard, a theory that supports politicized constructions of those with whom identifications via traumatic sufferings can be forged and those from whom such identifications are withheld" (Radstone 2007, p. 25).

By emphasizing the similarities between the individual traumatic experiences of the Oranienplatz protesters (before, during and after their flight to Germany) and the traumatic experiences of a range of people—fictional and other—whose lives most Germans would regard as valued, Erpenbeck attempts to establish empathy and shift these lives from ungrievable to grievable in Butler's terms. The narratives of refugees' suffering recounted by Erpenbeck have a "humanizing effect," producing "an intense identification by arousing feelings of fear and sorrow," much like the stories told in the media about the final moments of those who died in the World Trade Center, as discussed by Butler (Butler 2004, p. 38).

In the context of the current German refugee crisis, the philosopher Hilge Landweer confirmed the importance of drawing parallels to recognizable experiences for empathy to be felt, and emphasized

---

[9] Indeed, Hermes criticizes Erpenbeck for writing the traumatic experiences of the refugees in third person, as conveyed to Richard, and not from the first-person perspective of the refugees, yet such a first-person narrative would run the risk of both cultural appropriation and the appropriation of traumatic experiences (Hermes 2016, p. 185).

that empathy can be cultivated through a decided focus on commonalities and the belief that only luck is responsible for the fact that one is in a better situation (Landweer 2016). The focus on commonalities and similar personal or familial experiences is clear throughout *Gehen, ging, gegangen*, but Erpenbeck also emphasizes the role of fortune and the possibility that fortunes could be reversed. Noting that postwar posterity in Germany was not a result of the merits of individual Germans, Richard states, "[w]enn es aber nicht ihr eigenes Verdienst war, dass es ihnen so gut ging, war es andererseits auch nicht die Schuld der Flüchtlinge, dass es denen so schlecht ging" (Erpenbeck 2015, p. 120) ['[b]ut if this prosperity couldn't be attributed to their own personal merit, then by the same token the refugees weren't to blame for their reduced circumstances' (Erpenbeck 2017, chp. 19)]. Richard's friend Silvia, whose family also fled from the former Eastern territories, similarly reflects, "[i]ch stelle mir immer vor, dass auch wir noch einmal fliehen müssen, und dann wird uns auch niemand helfen" (Erpenbeck 2015, p. 120) ['I keep imagining that someday it'll be us having to flee, and no one will help us either' (Erpenbeck 2017, chp. 19)]. As all of the elements Landweer outlines work to awaken Richard's empathy for the refugees, it seems that Erpenbeck is simultaneously trying to awaken the same in the reader.

Erpenbeck's decision to make Richard a flawed and fallible individual, who describes the refugees as *kohlrabenschwarz* ['jet black'] (Erpenbeck 2015, p. 155), lusts after and objectifies the beautiful young woman of Ethiopian background who has volunteered to teach the protesters German (Erpenbeck 2015, pp. 134, 174),[10] and reflects over the course of the novel on the ways in which his treatment of his deceased wife was less than ideal, seems intended to make him and his experience of empathy with the asylum seekers identifiable to an imagined (fallible) German public. Indeed, the *Frankfurter Rundschau* review of *Gehen ging gegangen* went so far as to label Richard an everyman ('Jedermann') (Von Sternburg 2015), although the reviewer in *Die Welt* calls him 'kein Jedermann und kein Niemand' ['no everyman and no no-one'] (Lühmann 2015).[11] Yet, as Hermes notes, Richard's racism and naivety when it comes to matters of both cultural difference and refugee law decrease during the course of the novel as he gets to know the asylum seekers and familiarizes himself with the web of laws and regulations applying to them (Hermes 2016, p. 184).

6. Postmemory of the Flight from Silesia

Although Erpenbeck depicts a variety of Richard's personal experiences as leading to his growing empathy with the asylum seekers, including his continuing experience of disorientation and loss in post-reunification Berlin as an East Berliner, I will focus particularly on flight and expulsion. Since the beginning of the refugee crisis, a number of journalists, bloggers and other public commentators have reminded the public of the flight and expulsion of an estimated 12–14 million ethnic Germans from Central and Eastern Europe after World War II (Douglas 2012) (as compared to the arrival of a total of approximately 1.2 million asylum seekers in Germany between 2015 and 2016 (Drach 2017)). Memory of the flight and expulsions was a politically charged issue in Germany from the 1960s onwards, with memory politics divided along political lines. As Andreas Huyssen notes, "[t]he Right spoke of Dresden and the expulsion from the East, the Left spoke of Auschwitz" (Huyssen 2006, p. 184).[12] It is only in the years since reunification that remembering the expulsions and lost homes in the East has begun to be disentangled from revisionist and revanchist politics.[13] Most Germans have a personal

---

[10] A classics scholar lusting after a woman of Ethiopian descent has overtones of the colonialism that Richard criticizes elsewhere in the novel, first referring to the German colonization of Namibia (Erpenbeck 2015, p. 53), and later suggesting that the exploitative practices of Western companies in the current day suggest a continuation of colonialism (Erpenbeck 2015, p. 182).

[11] Alexandra Ludewig's suggestion that Richard is a *'Bildungsbürger'* [member of the educated classes] intended to represent a broad German middle class, is more persuasive (Ludewig 2016, p. 270).

[12] The left considered that the loss of the German lands was the price that the Germans had to pay for the atrocities of the Nazi-era, and that mourning this bereavement would only imply they did not understand their historical guilt.

[13] At the time of the turn of the millennium, the publication of a number of texts addressing or depicting German suffering during and after World War II—most prominently Jörg Friedrich's history of allied air raids on Germany from 1940–1945 *Der Brand* [*The Fire*], W G. Sebald's essay *Luftkrieg und Literatur* [*Air War and Literature*], and Günter Grass's novel *Im Krebsgang*

connection to the historical experience of flight and expulsion, as noted by Assmann, and this is one of the main reasons that supporters of Merkel's refugee policy have emphasized this history during the migrant crisis, hoping that these memories would help "*Ähnlichkeiten zu entdecken und Unterschiede zurückzustellen*" ['to discover similarities and to put aside differences'] (Assmann 2016b).

As Assmann notes elsewhere, Marianne's Hirsch term 'postmemory', which describes the transmission of traumatic experiences from one generation to the next, can be applied to the children of those ethnic Germans who fled or were expelled during and after World War II (Assmann 2016a). Hirsch writes:

> Postmemory characterizes the experience of those who grow up dominated by narratives that preceded their birth, whose own belated stories are evacuated by the stories of the previous generation shaped by traumatic events that can neither be understood nor recreated. I have developed this notion in relation to children of Holocaust survivors, but I believe it may usefully describe other second-generation memories of cultural or collective traumatic events and experiences (Hirsch 1997, p. 22).

Postmemory is *not* memory, "but at the same time, it approximates memory in its affective force" (Hirsch 2008, p. 109). Hirsch's concept of postmemory bears some relation to Landsberg's notion of prosthetic memory, which was developed more recently and was briefly discussed above, as both refer to the transmission of traumatic memories to someone who has never personally experienced the traumatic experience, but while Hirsch focuses on the transmission between family members over a long period of time, Landsberg envisions memories of traumatic events being transferred in contexts where there is no personal connection to the victims of those traumatic events.[14] The extent to which the narrative of Richard's mother's traumatic experiences dominated his childhood, and ingrained themselves in his memory, becomes clear in the following passage:

> *Er selbst war bei der Übersiedlung seiner Familie von Schlesien nach Deutschland noch ein Säugling gewesen und wäre im Tumult der Abreise beinahe von seiner Mutter getrennt worden, hätte ihn nicht auf dem überfüllten Bahnsteig ein russischer Soldat seiner Mutter über die Köpfe vieler anderer Aussiedler hinweg noch ins Zugabteil hineingereicht. Diese Geschichte war ihm von seiner Mutter so oft erzählt worden, dass er sie beinahe für seine eigene Erinnerung hielt* (Erpenbeck 2015, pp. 25–26).

> [He himself had been an infant when his family left Silesia and resettled in Germany. In the tumult of the departure, he almost got separated from his mother; he would have been left behind outright if it hadn't been for a Russian soldier, who, amid the press of the people on the station platform, handed him to his mother through the train's window over the head of many other resettlers.] (Erpenbeck 2017, chp. 3).

The traumatic transmitted memory of nearly being permanently separated from his mother has become almost indistinguishable from his own memory. This accords with Hirsch's description of postmemory as "the relationship of the second generation to powerful, often traumatic, experiences that preceded their births but were nevertheless *transmitted to them so deeply as to constitute memories*

[*Crabwalk*]—were widely hailed as signs that a taboo on German suffering in public discourse and literature had been lifted. While, as a number of commentators have since noted, it is inaccurate to speak of a previous blanket taboo on German suffering, the topic has since become much more widespread in German literature and public discourse and is no longer so tainted by association with right wing political groups (Stone 2016, pp. 19–20).

[14] Hirsch's concept of postmemory is also similar to LaCapra's notion of 'empathic unsettlement' discussed above, although the two theorists focus on different forms of the transmission of traumatic memory. Like LaCapra (LaCapra 2001, p. 40), Hirsch makes use of Kaja Silverman's concept of 'heteropathic identification' to posit a form of empathic connection that does not involve over-identification with, or appropriation of, the victim's experience (Hirsch 1997, p. 83). As Katherine Stone notes, "[t]he desire to bridge the gap between self and other, without unreflectively appropriating the latter's experiences, is for Hirsch a driving force of the work of postmemory" (Stone 2016, p. 475).

in their own rights" [emphasis added] (Hirsch 2008, p. 103). Richard's transferred memory deviates slightly from this description as he did experience the event directly, but at such a young age that it is extremely unlikely he would actually remember it. Elsewhere in the novel, Richard wonders whether his visceral reaction to the sound of a fire alarm siren at the refugee hostel is grounded in his own memory or transmitted memory: *"Richards Mutter hat mit ihm, er war noch ein Säugling, in einem Berliner Bombenkeller gesessen. Ob Richard sich an die Angst des Säuglings, der er war, oder an die Angst seiner Mutter erinnert? [...] Erinnert ein Säugling sich an den Krieg?"* (Erpenbeck 2015, pp. 214–15) ['Richard's mother had sat with him in a Berlin bomb cellar when he was just an infant. Can Richard remember the fear he felt as an infant, or his mother's fear? Can an infant remember a war? (Erpenbeck 2017, chp. 36)]. This postmemory also reminds him of the similarly traumatic memory of one of the refugees: *"Tristan hat gesagt: Wir saßen in den Baracken, als die europäischen Bomben auf Tripoli fielen, und hatten Angst, dass eine davon uns trifft"* (Erpenbeck 2015, p. 214) ['Tristan said once: We were sitting in the barracks when the European bombs fell over Tripoli and we were afraid one of them would hit us' (Erpenbeck 2017, chp. 36)]. A prosthetic memory has been formed, combining Tristan's narration of wartime Tripoli with Richard's "own archive of experience" (Landsberg 2004, p. 19). On the basis of his own postmemory and his prosthetic memory of wartime Tripoli, Richard can thus understand why one of the refugees, Yaya, cuts the wire for the siren, ending the *"mörderisch lauten Alarmton"* ['murderously loud alarm'], which is a form of *"Folter"* ['torture'], although he is not aware of the specific traumatic memory that leads Yaya to do so (Erpenbeck 2015, p. 214).

7. Conclusions

Both Assmann and Erpenbeck point out that the lack of empathy encapsulated in the xenophobia towards asylum seekers and other migrants in present-day Germany also has a precedent in the xenophobia encountered by the ethnic Germans arriving in postwar Germany from Central and Eastern Europe. Assmann notes the shocking parallels between xenophobia now and after World War II, when locals strengthened their sense of cohesion by discriminating against the refugees and the refugees encountered ridicule, abuse, and hateful slogans, some of which went so far as to suggest the refugees be sent to Auschwitz (Assmann 2016a). Richard is reminded by the rhyming slogan of an unnamed East German political party *"Lieber Geld für die Oma—als für Sinti und Roma"* ['Let's save our cash for Granny—not the Roma and Sinti'] and of Brecht's poem about a horse being eaten alive in post-World War I Berlin and worrying about the emotional calcification of its killers as it is being chopped apart (Erpenbeck 2015, p. 207; Erpenbeck 2017, chp. 34)[15]. Richard asks, *"[a]ber welchen Krieg hatten die Menschen jetzt hinter sich?"* (Erpenbeck 2015, p. 207) ['[b]ut what war have people now just been through?' (Erpenbeck 2017, chp. 34)], suggesting that there may have been understandable barriers to empathy in the deprivations of the immediate aftermath of World War I, but that these no longer exist.

Elsewhere in the novel, Richard also muses retrospectively that the tents on Oranienplatz were at risk of being set alight, implicitly alluding to the many arson attacks that have been made and continue to be made on refugee housing in Germany, especially in the East. He concludes: *"[d]ie Afrikaner wussten bestimmt überhaupt nicht, wer Hitler war, aber dennoch: Nur wenn sie Deutschland jetzt überlebten, hatte Hitler den Krieg wirklich verloren* (Erpenbeck 2015, p. 64) ['[t]he Africans probably had no idea who Hitler was, but even so: only if they survived Germany now would Hitler have lost the war' (Erpenbeck 2017, chp. 13)]. As Tyler notes, "[w]hile xenophobic discourses depict the asylum-seeker as a dehumanized, undifferentiated foreign mass, hoard [sic], influx, etc., humanitarian discourses ask the public to recognize 'the human face' of specific asylum-seekers" (Tyler 2006, p. 194). By telling the stories of the asylum seekers who occupied the Oranienplatz, Erpenbeck counters xenophobic

---

[15] Xenophobic attacks continue to be more common in the former GDR than elsewhere in Germany (Eckert 2017).

discourse and attempts to reposition the asylum seekers "as subjects who matter 'like us'" (Tyler 2006, p. 194), and bring them "under the rubric of the 'human'" (Butler 2004, p. 46).

Writing about the politics of literature, Jacques Ranciére explains that political activity "makes visible what was invisible, it makes audible as speaking beings those who were previously heard only as noisy animals" (Rancière 2011, p. 4), in other words the political work of literature is to expand points of emphatic connection.[16] Indeed, Ranciére's theory of politics as acts of becoming visible seems to be reflected in one of the slogans of the Oranienplatz protest mentioned a number of times in *Gehen, ging, gegangen*, "*we become visible.*"[17] In the novel, based on the interviews Erpenbeck herself held with the occupiers of Oranienplatz,[18] the lives of some members of the anonymous multitudes seeking refuge in Germany *do* become visible, *do* become grievable. By situating the current refugee crisis in the context of literary and historical experiences of displacement, and by focusing on individual stories of suffering, Erpenbeck overtly, but also successfully, appeals to the empathy of the reader. She reminds the reader of the commonalities of the traumatic experiences of the asylum seekers with the postwar flight and expulsion of ethnic Germans from Eastern Europe, a memory that many Germans share as either postmemory or prosthetic memory, and thus suggests, like Assmann, that "*unsere heutige Erfahrung der Migration verlangt nach einer längeren Perspektive, in der wir Zusammenhänge entdecken und Parallelen herstellen können*" ['our current experience of migration demands a longer perspective, in which we can discover coherencies and establish parallels'] (Assmann 2016a).

Conflicts of Interest: The author declares no conflict of interest.

References

Agamben, Giorgio. 1998. *Homo Sacer. Sovereign Power and Bare Life*. Translated by Daniel Heller-Roazen. Stanford: Stanford University Press.

Apel, Friedmar. 2015. Wir wurden, werden, sind sichtbar. *Die Frankfurter Allgemeine Zeitung*, September 16.

Assmann, Aleida. 2016a. Erinnerung an Flucht und Vertreibung nach dem Zweiten Weltkrieg. Available online: https://www.boell.de/de/2016/06/22/erinnerung-flucht-und-vertreibung-nach-dem-zweiten-weltkrieg (accessed on 29 May 2017).

Assmann, Aleida. 2016b. Hat Deutschland im Rahmen der Flüchtlingskrise eine besondere historisch bedingte Verantwortung? *Philosophie Magazin*, 48.

Assmann, Aleida, and Ines Detmers. 2016. *Empathy and Its Limits*. London: Palgrave Macmillan UK.

Bartels, Gerrits. 2015. Jenny Erpenbeck im Interview: 'Hinter der Ordnung verbirgt sich Angst.'. *Der Tagesspiegel*, October 12.

Bennett, Jill. 2005. *Empathic Vision: Affect, Trauma, and Contemporary Art*. Stanford: Stanford University Press.

Bhimji, Fazila. 2016. Visibilities and the Politics of Space: Refugee Activism in Berlin. *Journal of Immigrant and Refugee Studies*, 1–19. [CrossRef]

Buchzik, Dana. 2015. Trifft ein Berliner Professor auf Flüchtlinge. *Der Spiegel*, September 2.

Butler, Judith. 2004. *Precarious Life: The Powers of Mourning and Violence*. New York: Verso.

Craps, Stef. 2008. Linking Legacies of Loss: Traumatic Histories and Cross-Cultural Empathy in Caryl Phillips's *Higher Ground* and *The Nature of Blood*. *Studies in the Novel* 40: 191–202. [CrossRef]

Der Spiegel. 2017. Mehr als 3500 Angriffe auf Flüchtlinge. *Der Spiegel*, February 26.

Die Zeit. 2016. Zahl fremdenfeindlicher Attacken verdoppelt sich. *Die Zeit*, September 24.

Douglas, Ray M. 2012. *Orderly and Humane: The Expulsion of the Germans after the Second World War*. New Haven: Yale University Press.

---

[16] Both Landsberg and LaCapra also emphasize the potential for empathy to lead to social critique and political action (Landsberg 2004, p. 21; LaCapra 2001, p. 219).

[17] See also (Wilcke and Lambert 2015), which discusses the protests using Ranciére as a framework, but does not mention this slogan, cited by a number of news sources before the publication of the novel.

[18] In her acknowledgments Erpenbeck thanks thirteen males for "*viele gute Gespräche*" ('many good conversations') and also provides the account details for a charity that helps refugees in Berlin (Erpenbeck 2015, pp. 350–51).

Drach, Markus C. Schulte von. 2017. Zahl der Flüchtlinge in Deutschland extrem gesunken. *Süddeutsche Zeitung*, January 11.

Eagleton, Terry. 1970. *Exiles and Émigrés: Studies in Modern Literature*. London: Chatto & Windus.

Eckert, Daniel. 2017. Fremdenfeindlichkeit macht Ostdeutschland zum Risiko-Standort. *Die Welt*, March 17.

Erpenbeck, Jenny. 2015. *Gehen, ging, gegangen*. Munich: Knaus.

Erpenbeck, Jenny. 2017. *Go, Went, Gone*, Kindle ed. Translated by Susan Bernofsky. New York: New Directions.

Fadaee, Simin. 2015. The Immigrant Rights Struggle, and the Paradoxes of Radical Activism in Europe. *Social Movement Studies: Journal of Social, Cultural and Political Protest* 14: 733–39. [CrossRef]

Fieber, Marco. 2017. Die AfD sieht sich im Aufwind—Doch die Zahlen zeigen: Die Partei könnte an der 5-Prozent Hürde scheitern. *Huffington Post Germany*, April 28.

Gehrke, Christian. 2017. Gerhart-Hauptmann-Schule: Das kostet das Flüchtlingshaus wirklich. *Berliner Kurier*, May 22.

Goldberg, Amos. 2016. Empathy, Ethics, and Politics in Holocaust Historiography. In *Empathy and Its Limits*. Edited by Aleida Assmann and Ines Detmers. London: Palgrave Macmillan UK, pp. 52–76.

Hermes, Stefan. 2016. Grenzen der Repräsentation: Zur Inszenierung afrikanisch-europäischer Begegnungen in Jenny Erpenbecks Roman *Gehen, ging, gegangen*. *Acta Germanica: German Studies in Africa* 44: 171–91.

Hirsch, Marianne. 1997. *Family Frames: Photography, Narrative, and Postmemory*. Cambridge: Harvard University Press.

Hirsch, Marianne. 2008. The Generation of Postmemory. *Poetics Today* 29: 103–28. [CrossRef]

Huyssen, Andreas. 2006. Air War Legacies: From Dresden to Baghdad. In *Germans as Victims: Remembering the Past in Contemporary Germany*. Edited by Bill Niven. Basingstoke: Palgrave Macmillan, pp. 181–93.

LaCapra, Dominick. 2001. *Writing History, Writing Trauma*. Baltimore: Johns Hopkins University Press.

Landry, Olivia. 2015. "Wir sind alle Oranienplatz"! Space for Refugees and Social Justice in Berlin. *Seminar: A Journal of Germanic Studies* 51: 398–413. [CrossRef]

Landsberg, Alison. 2004. *Prosthetic Memory: The Transformation of American Remembrance in the Age of Mass Culture*. New York: Columbia University Press.

Landsberg, Alison. 2009. Memory, Empathy, and the Politics of Identification. *International Journal of Politics, Culture, and Society* 22: 221–29. [CrossRef]

Landsberg, Alison. 2015. *Engaging the Past: Mass Culture and the Production of Historical Knowledge*. New York: Columbia University Press.

Landweer, Hilge. 2016. Was sind die entscheidenden Faktoren dafür, dass wir Empathie mit Flüchtlingen empfinden? *Philosophie Magazin*, 47.

Ludewig, Alexandra. 2016. Jenny Erpenbecks Roman *Gehen, Ging, Gegangen* (2015). Eine zeitlose Odyssee und eine zeitspezifische Begebenheit. In *Niemandsbuchten und Schutzbefohlene: Flucht-Räume und Flüchtlingsfiguren in der Deutschsprachigen Gegenwartsliteratur*. Edited by Johannes Kleine and Charlton Payne Thomas Hardtke. Göttingen: V & R unipress, pp. 269–85.

Lühmann, Hannah. 2015. Ein Roman als Crashkurs in Flüchtlingskunde. *Die Welt*, August 31.

Magenau, Jörg. 2015. Ein Stückchen Acker in Ghana. *Die Süddeutsche Zeitung*, August 30.

Marciniak, Katarzyna, and Imogen Tyler. 2013. Immigrant Protest: An Introduction. *Citizenship Studies* 17: 143–56.

Nussbaum, Martha. 1995. *Poetic Justice: The Literary Imagination and Public Life*. Boston: Beacon.

Radstone, Susanna. 2007. Trauma Theory: Contexts, Politics, Ethics. *Paragraph* 30: 9–29. [CrossRef]

Rancière, Jacques. 2011. *The Politics of Literature*. Cambridge: Polity.

Said, Edward. 2002. *Reflections on Exile and Other Essays*. Cambridge: Harvard University Press.

Silverman, Kaja. 1996. *The Threshold of the Visible World*. New York: Routledge.

Sontag, Susan. 2007. Literature is Freedom. In *At the Same Time: Essays and Speeches*. Edited by Paolo Dilonardo and Anne Jump. New York: Farrar, Straus & Giroux, pp. 192–209.

Stockrahm, Sven. 2017. Je fremder, desto schlimmer unsere Fantasien. *Die Zeit*, February 8.

Stone, Brangwen. 2016. *Heimkehr? Narratives of Return to Germany's Former Eastern Territories 1965–2001*. Hannover: Wehrhahn Verlag.

Stone, Katherine. 2016. Sympathy, Empathy, and Postmemory: Problematic Positions in *Unsere Mütter, Unsere Väter*. *Modern Humanities Research Association* 111: 454–77.

Tyler, Imogen. 2006. "Welcome to Britain": The Cultural Politics of Asylum. *European Journal of Cultural Studies* 9: 185–202. [CrossRef]

UNHCR. 2017. UNHCR-Bericht: Flucht und Vertreibung erreichen 2016 neuen Höchstand. Available online: http://www.unhcr.org/dach/de/15212-globaltrends2016.html (accessed on 4 June 2017).

Von Sternburg, Judith. 2015. Jedermann und die Afrikaner. *Frankfurter Rundschau*, September 1.

Wiedemann, Caroline. 2015. Was wurde aus den Aktivisten vom Oranienplatz? *Der Spiegel*, April 22.

Wilcke, Holger, and Laura Lambert. 2015. Die Politik des O-Platzes. (Un)Sichtbare Kämpfe einer Geflüchteten Bewegung. *Movements: Journal für kritische Migrations-und Grenzregimeforschung*, vol. 1. Available online: http://movements-journal.org/issues/02.kaempfe/06.wilcke,lambert--oplatz-k%C3%A4mpfe-gefl%C3%BCchtete-bewegung.html (accessed on 22 July 2017).

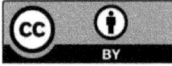

humanities

MDPI

Article

Post-Dictatorship Documentary in Chile: Conversations with Three Second-Generation Film Directors

Antonio Traverso

School of Media, Creative Arts and Social Inquiry, Curtin University, Bentley 6102, Australia;
a.traverso@curtin.edu.au

Received: 28 November 2017; Accepted: 9 January 2018; Published: 14 January 2018

Abstract: No other medium has rejected the restorative narrative of Chile's democratic state's memory discourse as vigorously as documentary cinema. After the several democratic governments that succeeded the civic-military dictatorial alliance that ruled this nation uninterruptedly between 1973 and 1990, documentary films have resisted monumental versions of historical memory by confronting the ambivalent nuances of the traumatic legacy of the dictatorship. Chilean documentarians have investigated, uncovered, and depicted the dictatorial state's crimes, while offering testimonial space to survivors, and have also interrogated the perspectives of the dictatorship's supporters, collaborators, and perpetrators while wrestling with an open dialectic of confrontational and reconciliatory gestures. More recently, this interest has intensified and combined with what is often described as a "boom" in second-generation personal-narration memory films. The present article includes the author's conversations with the directors of three recent Chilean second-generation documentaries that explore the perspectives of former secret service collaborators: Adrian Goycoolea's ¡*Viva Chile Mierda!* [*Long Live Chile, Damn It!*] (2014), Andrés Lübbert's *El color del camaleón* [*The Color of the Chameleon*] (2017), and Lissette Orozco's *El pacto de Adriana* [*Adriana's Pact*] (2017).

Keywords: documentary; Chile; dictatorship; Pinochet; torture; trauma; memory; perpetrators; post-conflict; reconciliation

1. Introduction

Chile's process of transitional justice after General Pinochet's alliance with the Chilean economic civilian elite that ruled this country through an uninterrupted dictatorial regime between 1973 and 1990 has been entrapped within a prescriptive, state-sponsored restorative notion of national reconciliation, highly reliant on perpetrators' impunity and vigorously rejected by survivors and their supporters. Critics of the official reconciliation discourse in this nation have instead directed their attention to Chile's highly productive grass-roots memory culture—which includes independent journalism, social research, memory sites, literature, performance, music, and visual and screen arts—giving preference to agonistic concepts of social reconciliation. Arguably, no other medium has rejected the reductionist, restorative narrative of the democratic state's memory discourse as unwaveringly and vigorously as Chilean documentary cinema. Documentary films have resisted monumental versions of historical memory by confronting the painfully ambivalent, incomplete, and at times contradictory nuances of the traumatic legacy of the dictatorship. While the majority of the documentaries made in Chile after the end of the dictatorship naturally sought to denounce crimes against humanity, centering their attention on historical narration, forensic and legal investigation, depiction of evidence, and survivor testimony, two landmark films were the first to open up to the exploration of the perspective of former secret service collaborators: *La Flaca Alejandra* [*Skinny Alexandra*] (1994), directed by Carmen Castillo and Guy Girard (Castillo and Girard 1994), which focuses on a conversation with a former revolutionary who after her arrest and subsequent torture went on to become an agent of the secret service, and *El mocito* [*The Young Butler*] (2011), directed by Marcela Said and Jean de Certau (Said and de Certau 2011), which centers on the testimony of a man who as a teenager was employed as an errand boy at one of the dictatorship's torture houses. More recently, the interest in the figures of the dictatorship's supporter, collaborator, and perpetrator has intensified with what can be described as a "boom" in second-generation personal-narration memory documentaries in Chile and in other Latin American post-conflict societies.

The present article includes the edited text of the author's recent conversations with the directors of three second-generation documentaries, namely, Adrian Goycoolea's *¡Viva Chile Mierda!* [*Long Live Chile, Damn It!*] (2014), Andrés Lübbert's *El color del camaleón* [*The Color of the Chameleon*] (2017), and Lissette Orozco's *El pacto de Adriana* [*Adriana's Pact*] (2017). All people interviewed agreed to participate and for their names and email addresses to be provided in the article. In the first film, Goycoolea explores the reconciliation of his aunt and uncle with a former agent of Pinochet's secret police who guarded them when they were prisoners at an interrogation and torture center in Santiago in the early 1970s. In the second film, Lübbert confronts and reconciles with his father, who in 1978 escaped from Chile to seek refuge in Europe after being abducted, tortured, and forced to undertake intelligence and repressive training with the secret service. Finally, in *El pacto de Adriana*, Orozco confronts her aunt, a former agent of Pinochet's secret police, who is sought by the Chilean courts on charges of collaboration in several cases of kidnapping, torture, and murder. As can be appreciated in the interviews that follow, these recent second-generation, post-dictatorship Chilean documentaries are prime examples of the ongoing interrogation of the perspective of the dictatorship's collaborator, as their directors grapple with the shifting, problematic, and interrelated dynamics of confrontation and reconciliation.

2. Adrian Goycoolea's *¡Viva Chile Mierda!*

Adrian Goycoolea (Figure 1) was born in Brazil to Chilean and British parents and has lived in Brazil, Chile, the US, and the UK. He finished high school in 1991 and then completed one year of an audiovisual communication degree at UNIACC (University of Arts, Science and Communication) in Santiago, Chile. Between 1993 and 1997, he studied filmmaking at New York's School of Visual Arts and then worked as a programmer and publicist at Anthology Film Archives and in various capacities at MoMA, Hollywood.com, and *The New York Times*. In 2003, Goycoolea started a Master of Fine Arts (MFA) at the University of Iowa, and in 2007, he moved to the UK, where he is currently Senior Lecturer in Film Studies at the University of Sussex. His screen work ranges from experimental film and personal documentary to multi-channel installations, addressing issues of location, identity, memory, and political histories. *¡Viva Chile Mierda!*, written and directed by Goycoolea, is the director's first feature-length documentary.[1]

---

[1]   Director's Email: A.P.Goycoolea@sussex.ac.uk

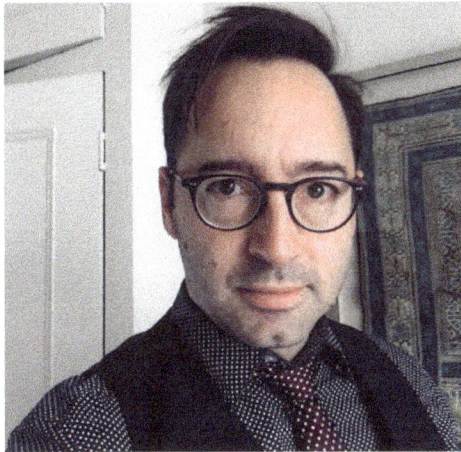

Figure 1. Director Adrian Goycoolea. Picture courtesy of Adrian Goycoolea.

Structured as a personal narration through Goycoolea's reflexive voiceover, *¡Viva Chile Mierda!* (Figure 2) includes a series of highly significant interviews, such as an original conversation with former agent of Pinochet's secret police Andrés Valenzuela. Valenzuela, who defected from the service in the early 1980s, provided vital information about the pernicious practices of the repressive apparatus, including details concerning missing detainees, to Chilean journalist Mónica González, who is also interviewed in the film. Goycoolea's documentary features additional conversations between the director and his aunt Gaby, who, not long after the coup of 1973, was held prisoner along with her husband in a torture center in Santiago, where they were guarded by Valenzuela, their former neighbor. In the film, Goycoolea also talks with his cousins in their home in Spain, who revisit together their traumatic memories of being raided by soldiers in their Santiago home, witnessing their parents' being taken away, and then being forced into a life in exile. Goycoolea's film explores the reconciliation of his aunt and uncle with Valenzuela. *¡Viva Chile Mierda!* has screened internationally, including New York, Santiago, Geneva, Rijeka, Glasgow, Madrid, Barcelona, and Brighton. It was listed as one of the ten best Chilean films of 2014 by Twitchfilm.com.

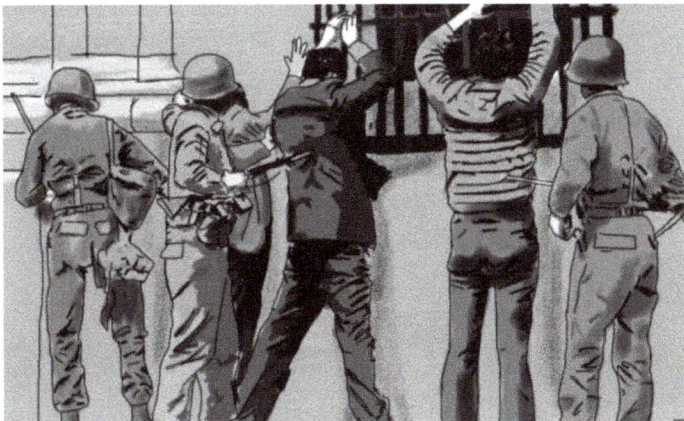

Figure 2. Frame from *¡Viva Chile Mierda!* (Goycoolea 2014). Picture courtesy of Adrian Goycoolea.

Antonio Traverso (AT): Do you identify as Chilean?[2]

Adrian Goycoolea (AG): I do consider myself Chilean, but given that I grew up in Brazil, the US, and Chile, I have a somewhat conflicted sense of national identity. I suppose I'm something of a Pan-American subject.

AT: When did you decide to make a documentary about your family's story?

AG: The idea came to me when I found out about the unexpected reunion between my uncle, Sergio Córdova, and Andrés Valenzuela in Spain around 2005. Soon after I moved to the UK to take up my post at the University of Sussex in 2007, my Uncle Sergio told me the full story when I visited him, my Aunt Gaby, and my cousins in their home in Spain. My uncle died the following year. I thought it was an incredible story for a documentary, so I began filming in 2010.

AT: What response did you get from your family?

AG: I knew it would be difficult for them to speak on camera about what they had been through. I was particularly nervous about approaching my Aunt Gaby. Much to my surprise, she said that the timing was perfect. She and her children had had to write down their experiences for the bid they were submitting to the Chilean government to receive reparations. They hadn't discussed it as a family yet, and she thought that my film might be a good opportunity to do it. It still wasn't easy for them. My cousin Ximena, the youngest sibling, ended up calling me on the day of the interview to tell me that she had left the house to come to the shoot only to turn around and go back home because she simply couldn't do it. My cousin Sergio Cristian (Chacal), the second younger sibling, also found it very difficult, and it was touch and go whether or not he would be able to go through with the interview. We actually started the conversation without him, but after a while, he joined the group and shared his experiences.

AT: How did journalist Mónica González respond?

AG: Mónica González was incredibly warm and accommodating. What sparked her interest was my telling her that I had recently interviewed Andrés Valenzuela. She had not heard from him—no one had—since he left Chile after her unprecedented interview with him in 1984. So, she must have been curious to hear what Valenzuela had said to me. It's likely that her conversation with me may have been the first time she spoke on camera and in such detail about her experience with Valenzuela in the 1980s.

AT: How did you find and get to interview Valenzuela?

AG: The main problem was that not even his close friends had a means of contacting Valenzuela directly. They would only communicate with him when he was in touch with them and this was sporadic. Through my contacts among Chilean exiles, I sent him an interview request in 2011. Some months later, I heard back that he wasn't interested. I tried to contact him directly, but I hit a brick wall. None of his friends had heard from him in months, and they were reluctant to relay new messages from me. But I hadn't given up hope to find a way to speak with him. From my conversations with Valenzuela's friends, I had a hunch he might be working for a certain company in France, which, unfortunately, had branches all over France, and I had no way of knowing where to start. I memorized how to say in French: "Hello, I'm looking for Andrés Valenzuela, does he work here?" and off I went to France with a list of addresses in the summer of 2011. Luckily, I hit the jackpot the first place I went to, and somebody pointed him out to me. When I approached him with my single French sentence, he replied also in French: "Yes, I'm Andrés Valenzuela". I then switched to Spanish

2   Interview conducted via email in 2016–2017. Goycoolea provided answers in English, which I subsequently edited. He reviewed earlier drafts and approved the final version of the interview. I thank him for his interest and support and for providing me with photographs, media materials, and access to his film.

and explained who I was. He hurriedly asked me to come back after work, adding that we should talk elsewhere. I was anxious that he might not be there when I returned, but he was, and he agreed to be interviewed. Probably, it helped that I said that the focus of my film was his relationship with my aunt and uncle, toward whom he felt warmly. We drove to a nearby restaurant, where I shot the video interview. When we finished, he told me that had I approached him in Spanish, he would have said he didn't know who Andrés Valenzuela was. But because I looked like a *gringo* and spoke rubbish French, he had no reason to think I was Chilean. He also told me that he had not wanted to be interviewed before because he had been considering traveling to Chile to visit his family and didn't want to be back in the public consciousness, hoping that he'd been forgotten and it was safe to go back. But a short time before I found him, a popular Chilean television drama series was aired that had a character based on him. So, he felt that his plans of returning to Chile had already been dashed and he might as well be interviewed by me.

AT: Have you stayed in contact with Valenzuela?

AG: When I was in Chile for the premiere of my film at the International Documentary Festival of Santiago (FIDOCS) in 2014, I found out that Valenzuela had recently been in the country visiting his family. Possibly because of the time lag between our interview in France and my film's premiere in Chile, he might have thought it was safe for him to go back. I was glad to know that he'd finally returned home. I also learned that while he was there, he'd been summoned by a Chilean judge to testify in court for several human rights cases that had been launched as a result of his original "confession" to Mónica González in 1984. I hope that his testimony was useful to the Chilean court. I had no contact with Valenzuela for quite a while after our interview in 2011. I couldn't even send him a copy of the film, since he had stopped working for that French company. I wasn't even sure if he knew that I had completed the film. But recently, we got in touch via Facebook. He told me that he had seen my film and that he found it "very moving and well made" and that it made him "travel back in time".

AT: How did the Chilean public and media respond to the film?

AG: I was anxious to see how the film would be received in Chile given that I speak in English with an American accent and also because of my film's sympathetic treatment of Valenzuela. But in the Questions and Answers (Q&A) session many in the audience said they had been moved by the film. Some of them told their own stories, quite similar to my family's. Some had traumatic experiences at the hands of the secret service but had never told their families. There were stories of families divided across political lines. Media reviews tended to center on my interview with Valenzuela. This is not surprising in view of the fact that images of Valenzuela had not been seen on Chilean screens since he'd left the country almost thirty years earlier. My film is now permanently housed at the Museum of Memory and Human Rights in Santiago, where it screens occasionally and is available through their Center of Audiovisual Documentation. A few months after the premiere in Chile, my film was shown in Geneva, where the audience consisted mostly of Chilean exiles and their families. In the Q&A session, many people conveyed how moved they were by my aunt's testimony and the way the film approaches the experience of exile.

AT: What was it like for you to make this film?

AG: Making this film was a long, difficult process. It involved traveling from the UK to Spain, France, and Chile between 2010 and 2013. Fortunately, I had support from the University of Sussex, where I teach filmmaking, to cover travel expenses to shoot interviews. With no other resources, I did pretty much everything: production, directing, camera, editing, animation. There were only a few interviews in which I had someone helping me with the sound recorder, and the final sound mix was done professionally by a cousin of mine, Nadine Voullieme Uteau, in Chile. The scene in which my cousins have a conversation around the table in my aunt's kitchen was very difficult to film as I didn't have anyone to help me with the sound. To shoot that scene, I engineered an extendable arm that

I attached onto my camera so that I could re-position the shotgun microphone while still not being in the shot. This made the video camera heavier and more cumbersome, which caused me to have some issues with image stability and mic noise. I was dripping with sweat after that shoot, since I was filming handheld for over two hours straight. But, shooting by myself this way allowed for a far greater level of intimacy with my family. I also used different recording formats. For example, there is a sequence towards the end of the film in which I shot my aunt and cousins at Park Güell with a Super-8 film camera. I decided to use Super-8 in this scene to present a different aesthetic of memory: the home movie, which is coded both as nostalgia and as a source of documentary evidence for a familial narrative. This sequence directly precedes the semi-final scene of the film, which shows actual home video footage of my aunt and uncle visiting their old haunts in Papudo, Chile, several years ago. For me, these two sequences highlight the way in which the aggregation of family memories proceeds to form cultural and historical narratives that we retell in order to create a coherent sense of self, both as individuals and as nations. ¡*Viva Chile Mierda!* is my first feature-length film, and as such, it marks a turning point in my career in terms of scope and ambition. It is also the most complex subject I have tackled thus far. I believe that I am getting closer to finding my personal voice, especially in terms of how best to mix the personal with the political.

AT: Is this a first-person film?

AG: When I was planning my film, I had in mind the films of Patricio Guzmán, Chris Marker, Agnes Varda, and Jonas Mekas in connection with first-person documentary approaches, especially in terms of the use of the device of the personal voice over. But I suppose I didn't include footage of myself on camera in the way other Chilean memory documentarians have done because this wasn't really my life's story. I also thought that by asking the interview questions myself as well as filming, editing and narrating the film, there was already enough of my presence. Without removing myself entirely, I was trying to leave as much room as I could to my subjects.

AT: Why do you use animation in your film?

AG: My decision to use animation responded to practical and conceptual factors. One practical reason was that much of my family's photographic archive had been confiscated by the military when my aunt was detained. The second problem was that I didn't have the funds to pay for archival material. So, by transforming archival photographs of the coup into drawings, I no longer needed to pay for the rights. More importantly, I was able to represent well-trodden historical images in a new light, thereby personalizing the historical archive. I feel that the archival imagery of the 1973 coup has been seen by the Chilean public so much that it has lost some of its impact. I felt that by drawing it in a simple way, I could render it both more accessible and more affecting, because of the tension between the naive aesthetic and the traumatic nature of the historical footage. Also, in a more general sense, I am interested in the nature of memory as it relates to the creation of historical narratives. This is why I animated the drawing of some of the images as a way to indicate that memory—and by extension, history—is an act of creation. Every time we remember something we recreate it in our minds. The drawings in my film, although based on the photographic archive, are my interpretation of these indexical images. This seems like an important metaphor when dealing with historical material in a documentary context. Some of the pictures of my family, in particular the "photograph" of Valenzuela with his arm around my Uncle Sergio, are fabrications that create images of events for which there is no photographic record.

3. Andrés Lübbert's *El color del camaleón*

Andrés Lübbert (Figure 3) was born in Belgium in 1985 to a Belgian mother and a Chilean father. He completed a Master's degree in Audiovisual Arts at Brussels' Royal Arts School in 2010. His documentaries have participated in more than 140 film festivals in 20 countries, winning close to 30 prizes. Lübbert's films address themes of interculturalism, migration, identity, human rights, and social issues. His short documentary *The Reality* (Lübbert 2009) was nominated for the Golden Key at the Kassel Documentary Film Festival in Germany, and, in 2013, he was Vocation Award laureate in Belgium for his commitment to social documentary filmmaking. He directed the short fiction film *Fistful of Memories* (Lübbert 2014) about Turkish and Moroccan migration to Antwerp and the documentary *Dying for Life* (Lübbert 2016) about a Syrian refugee in Belgium. Written and directed by Lübbert, *El color del camaleón* (Lübbert 2017) is the director's first feature-length documentary.[3]

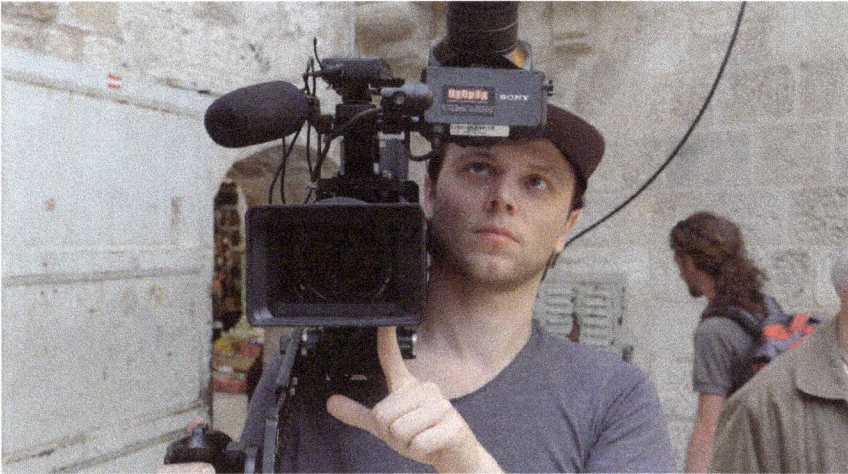

Figure 3. Director Andrés Lübbert. Picture courtesy of Andrés Lübbert.

El color del camaleón (Figure 4) is a personal-narration documentary in which the director appears on screen to confront his father, Chilean-born war reporter Jorge Lübbert. In 1978, in the midst of Chile's dictatorship, Lübbert's father, then a twenty-one-year-old technical drawing graduate, who had recently started a job with the state-owned telephone company, was kidnapped and taken hostage by the secret service, being released and abducted consecutively over a period of five months. Forced to collaborate through torture and death threats, he was trained to perform intelligence and repressive work. Psychologically crushed, the director's father fled Chile later that year, seeking asylum in the former East Germany and then in Belgium, where he eventually got married and fathered two sons, the youngest being Andrés. In the film, the director poses questions to his father about his past in Chile, the reasons for his exile, and the cause of his traumatic symptoms, which Lübbert witnessed as he grew up. Narratively structured through the director's reflexive voiceover, the film deviates from the conventional first-person narration of recent memory documentaries to adopt a second-person address through which Lübbert appears to talk to his father. In the film, father and son are seen traveling together from their Belgian home to Chile, where they share a trajectory of traumatic memory, visiting former torture centers and ultimately allowing a reconciliatory dialogue to open up between them. *El color del camaleón* premiered at SANFIC (International Film Festival of Santiago) in August 2017, where it won the Best Director and the Public's awards. The film has screened widely, including venues in Argentina, Belgium, Bulgaria, Chile, Ecuador, Germany, Mexico, and Perú.

---

[3] Director's Email: andreslubbert@hotmail.com

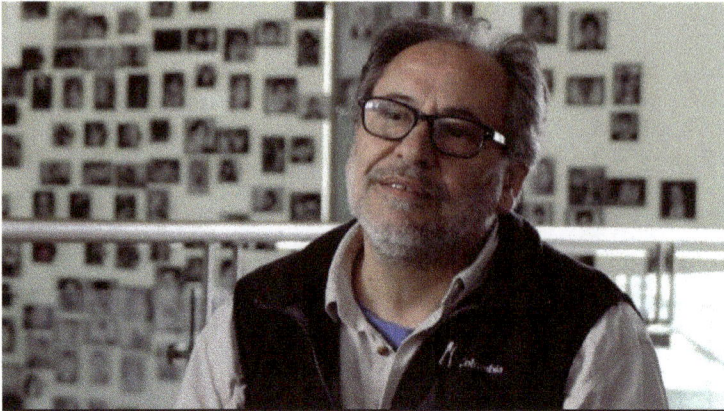

Figure 4. Jorge Lübbert, pictured; frame from *El color del camaleón* (Lübbert 2017). Picture courtesy of Andrés Lübbert.

AT: How did you learn Spanish?[4]

Andrés Lübbert (AL): When I was a child, my father refused to speak Spanish at home. So, we spoke Flemish. When I was about nineteen, I traveled to Chile for the first time. Since I didn't speak Spanish, I half-communicated in English and sign language. Later, I studied Spanish grammar in Madrid and then traveled throughout Latin America. When I got back home to Belgium, I forced my father to speak Spanish with me.

AT: How did you get into filmmaking?

AL: I never thought of becoming a filmmaker when I was younger; it happened almost by chance. I actually wanted to be a professional soccer player. I used to be as obsessed with soccer as I am now with cinema. While traveling, I made two documentaries without having studied film, let alone thinking of it as a profession. But soon after, I discovered the cinema of Argentina, which had a huge impact on me, especially the realist films of the New Argentine Cinema. I then started to think seriously about filmmaking, and, in 2005, I enrolled for one year at Universidad del Cine, Argentina, after which I spent about four years completing a Master's degree in audiovisual arts in Brussels. Before *El color del camaleón*, I made fifteen documentaries, but they were no-budget films in which I worked on my own or sometimes with just one more person. *El color del camaleón* is the first film for which I had a production budget and a full professional crew.

AT: What was this transition like for you?

AL: With a budget and professional assistance, I spent more time redrafting the script, designing the visual style, and planning the shoots. Earlier, I'd made my films quickly, some in one or two weeks. Although there is something special about working fast, I don't think I gave those films as much thought as I should have. But going from working on my own to working with a team of professionals

---

4   I conducted an informal video conversation with Lübbert in person and in Spanish in Santiago, Chile, on 4 September, 2017. On the same occasion, Chilean media producers Rodrigo Gonçalves and Fernando Villagrán conducted a formal video interview with Lübbert, also in Spanish, for *Off the Record*, a Chilean cultural program nearly two decades old, created and produced independently for Chilean television. I thank Gonçalves and Villagrán for giving me permission to videotape and use their interview (*Off the Record*'s and my questions are respectively marked with initials here). I subsequently transcribed, translated into English, and edited Lübbert's responses, and he reviewed earlier drafts and approved the final version of the full interview. I thank him for his interest and support and for providing me with photographs, media materials, and access to his film.

wasn't difficult for me at all because I'm good at giving instructions. As a soccer player, I used to be extremely competitive, and, often, I was my team's captain. It wasn't hard to transfer these skills to my filmmaking. In my previous films, I performed most of the creative roles myself. I don't think I like one function more than any other. I enjoy the thinking and the writing at the beginning, but I also love going on shoots and the post-production.

AT: Why did you shift the first-person narration of recent post-dictatorship documentaries to a second-person address in your film?

AL: This film started as my attempt to open a dialogue with my father. This desire eventually became the film's central narrative conflict. As you see it from the start of the film, I speak to my father without getting a response from him. So, it was clear to me that the narration had to be structured through my voiceover and that it had to be addressed to my father. I had done voiceover narrations in some of my previous films but never in this way. This "speaking to my father" narrative structure also means that my father eventually came to share his most personal secret with me and at the same time with everybody else. Since my father works in the film and television industry, he was always very aware when I was filming him and of what everybody would see and hear. So, in the end, he not only tells me his hidden story but also trusts me to choose what I make public and how. My father's trust in me ultimately becomes a demonstration of his love for me.

AT: Do you expect your father to make his own film in response to yours?

AL: No, it is enough that in my film he eventually answers me. We shared very intense experiences travelling together to Palestine, Germany, and Chile. We are much closer to each other now, and this is what making the film was for in the first place: that he and I would be able to talk. My father said that making this film helped him to open his heart.

AT: Were you expecting the kind of public response your film had in Chile?

AL: I've been very surprised by it. It's been like a dream. I won the Best Director and the Public's awards at SANFIC 2017, and after the screenings, people showed me great affection and gratitude. I saw them queue to share with me their own experiences during the dictatorship. Never before had anything this special happened to me.

Off The Record (OTR): What does the film's title mean?

AL: The "chameleon" of the title symbolizes my father. So, in the film, I'm asking what his real color is. As a child, an obsession grew in me to find out who my father was. I saw him suffer from depression, insomnia, addictions, but I didn't understand why. I witnessed his self-destructive behavior, going to conflict zones as a reporter for more than thirty years. He literally traveled around the world seeking mortal danger. I imagined an idealized friendship with him that I didn't have. I made this film to find out who my father was and, ultimately, also who I was.

OTR: When did you first approach your father?

AL: I started to wonder about my own identity at around nineteen. I had never been in Chile, and I decided to come here. I learned some Spanish, met my Chilean family, and made my first documentary, *My Father, My Story*. In that film, I tell the story of my father in a very naïve way. I didn't know much about the dictatorship, so I interviewed some of my relatives and people who work in human rights. I began to get personally entangled in this story, which to me was very difficult to understand. It was like a great jigsaw puzzle for which I had many disconnected pieces. I went back to Belgium without any answers about what had happened to my father in Chile. My filmmaker uncle, Orlando Lübbert, told me that when my father escaped from Chile and then went from East Germany to Belgium, he started treatment with psychotherapist Jorge Barudy, who in those days had created a support center for exiled Latin American torture victims. In therapy, my father began a process of reparation through the reconstruction of his personal history. The first thing he did in therapy was to record his testimony on audiotape, which my Uncle Orlando later transcribed. When I was twenty-two, my uncle gave me the full transcript to read, in which my dad describes in the first person what happened to him in Chile. I actually use parts of this very intense testimony in my film. But, at the time, I didn't know what to do with that dense document, so, in order to understand it, I began a search to confirm the facts in it. I needed to understand that awfully harsh history that was rather unknown to me. At first, I wanted to talk with my father about it, but I knew he suffered from a deep trauma. I could perceive his pain, so I didn't have the courage to ask him anything for some time. One day, I spoke to him when we were together on a long drive in Belgium. However, I only asked him one question about his past, and he was unable to say a single word. I realized that his trauma was too deep, the memory of his experiences too painful, so I let it go. Only after some years, when I had finished my Master's degree in filmmaking, did I decide to return to this story. I proposed to my father to reconstruct his past by making a film with me. He agreed. I don't think he did it for himself, other people, or Chile. He did it for me, because he could see that I was suffering too.

OTR: What was it like for you and your father to shoot the film together in Chile?

AL: Although it took only four months, it was a life-changing process for my father. Thanks to it, he managed to break through his inability to speak about his past in Chile. The hardest was when we visited places where he'd been through terrible experiences. As a child, I used to see my dad going to war zones for his work and never showing any fear. He was taken prisoner by the Taliban in Afghanistan, by guerrillas in El Salvador, and by Blackwater Security in Iraq, and he always survived. He was as strong as a rock. But in Chile, I saw a fear in him I'd never seen before. It was puzzling to see terror in his eyes, to see him out of breath or become paralyzed with paranoia when we visited certain locations. I could sense his pain and fear, and it was very hard for me to see him like that. But I think I was also able to cure in great measure the trauma he had passed on to me. This is why the film is constructed as a dialogue about the past between my father and me. You can see that my father wants to answer my questions but finds it extremely difficult to do so. Progressively, he is able to open up and reconnect with his past. Shooting the film together was a healing experience for both of us, and as a result, we also became much closer than before.

OTR: How was your father affected by his participation in the film?

AL: I think it took a huge load off him. This doesn't mean that my father got rid of his terror. Probably, he is always going to have this fear within him. To give you an example: during the process of production, I collected many documents with information about military personnel in order to have evidence that they had been members of the secret service. By the end of the production, I had two large piles of such documents, some of which didn't even make it into the film. Before returning to Belgium, my father forced me to dissolve in water all this paperwork in order to eliminate any traces of what we had done. He didn't want anybody finding in the rubbish proof that we had been making the film. He said that those who were in the secret service before still had considerable power in Chile. Although I could perceive that his fear was real, I myself wasn't afraid at all, and I dismissed his concerns. I acknowledge that sometimes I may have approached the film's production in a rather naïve way. As someone from a younger generation, born overseas and not having gone through a dictatorship, I simply thought that we needed to tell this story and couldn't see anything of which to be frightened.

OTR: How was your interaction with audiences after screenings in Chile?

AL: Before the film premiered at SANFIC we had avant-premieres at five Chilean universities. Since we knew that it is difficult to attract young people to documentary screenings, we decided to take the film to them. Audience reactions were diverse but all rather intense. After the screenings at SANFIC, I must have received hundreds of hugs from very emotional people, not only torture victims but also children of victims and even children of perpetrators. There was one woman, the daughter of a general charged with crimes against humanity, who approached me in tears, saying that the film had deeply touched her. Ultimately, the children and grandchildren of the perpetrators of the dictatorship did not have a choice in what their parents and grandparents did. But they also became part of the same collective trauma and culture of silence with respect to the past. Perhaps films like mine can help to start a dialogue between young Chileans and the generation who experienced the dictatorship.

OTR: Do you see Chileans as a society either addressing or avoiding this conversation?

AL: My father's personal history, with his trauma and amnesia, is typical of what has been happening with the country at large. With the return to democracy in 1990, most Chileans avoided thinking about the past and sought to move on. Only after so many years it is becoming possible to heal from the wounds of the past through reflection, dialogue, and remembrance. What I see in Chile from the outside is a clear-cut divide between political opposites. But in my father's story, we can see that history is neither black nor white but multicolored. This is why it's important to open up to different kinds of dialogue and different versions of history. My film proposes the idea that, through inter-generational dialogue, it may be possible to come together as a society. Documentaries like mine also constitute valuable documents for future generations. When those who were direct witnesses of the dictatorship have passed, who is going to keep their memory alive so that these terrible events do not take place again? My film conveys a message of hope for the future, but now we need to take a step aside and let the younger generation speak.

4. Lissette Orozco's *El pacto de Adriana*

Lissette Orozco (Figure 5) was born in Santiago, Chile, in 1987. She studied audiovisual communication, specializing in film and television screenwriting, and completed a Master's degree in documentary cinema at Santiago's UNIACC (University of Arts, Science and Communication) in 2011. Orozco has taught at UNIACC and Diego Portales University and worked as a freelance researcher, scriptwriter, assistant director, and director in independent documentary production and in docureality shows for public television in Chile. She wrote and directed the award-winning short documentaries *El día ideal* [*The Ideal Day*] (Orozco 2010), *Subsuelo* [*Underground*] (Orozco 2014), and *Vorágine* [*Vortex*] (Orozco 2014), as well as the multiple-award-winning feature-length documentary *El pacto de Adriana* [*Adriana's Pact*] (Orozco 2017). As assistant director, Orozco is currently completing a documentary about the Chilean writer and performer Pedro Lemebel. Orozco migrated to Bogotá, Colombia, in 2017, where she teaches documentary at the National Film School and continues to work as project advisor, scriptwriter, and independent documentary director.[5]

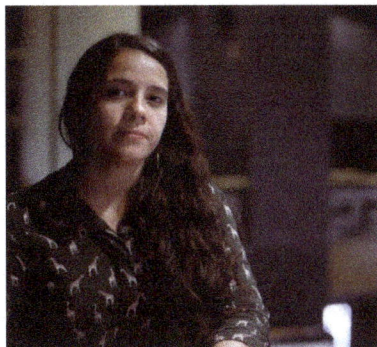

Figure 5. Director Lissette Orozco. Picture courtesy of Lissette Orozco.

---

[5]   Director's Email: liss.orozco@gmail.com

Lissette Orozco's aunt, Adriana Rivas, migrated to Australia in the 1970s. As a result, the director of *El pacto de Adriana* (Figure 6) always knew her as "Aunty Chany from Australia," who would visit every now and then and stay at her home in Santiago for a month. In 2007, Rivas was arrested by Chilean police as she attempted to go through customs at Santiago's international airport on one of her routine visits. Thus begins Orozco's search to find out about her aunt's past, to which she had been largely oblivious until then. Initially, she collected news items about her aunt's case while keeping a video journal, but in 2011, when she was completing a Master's degree in filmmaking, Orozco launched the production of a full documentary, *El pacto de Adriana*. Orozco learned that her aunt had been an agent of the National Intelligence Directorate (DINA), Pinochet's notorious secret service, in the early 1970s, and that she was being charged with collaboration in several cases of kidnapping, torture, and murder. However, the same year that Orozco started her film, Adriana Rivas, who had been released on parole with a prohibition to leave the country, secretly escaped from Chile and returned to her home in Sydney, where she still lives. The film narrates Orozco's trajectory in the interaction with her aunt, moving from trust to suspicion and from the desire for reconciliation to confrontation, public exposé, and total family rupture. *El pacto de Adriana* screened in more than forty international film festivals in 2017, receiving over ten prizes, including the Peace Award at the 2017 Berlin International Film Festival. It was also nominated for the Phoenix Awards in 2017.

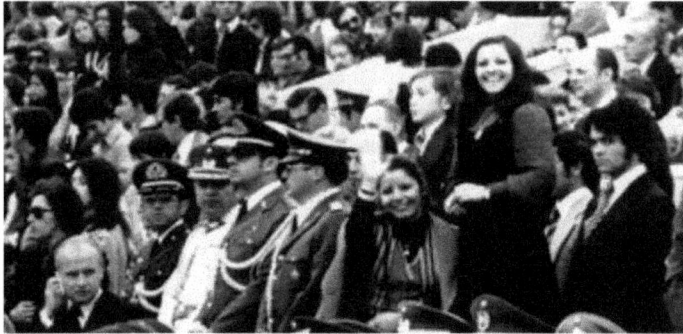

Figure 6. Adriana Rivas, pictured waving, in the early 1970s; frame from *El pacto de Adriana* (Orozco 2017). Picture courtesy of Lissette Orozco.

AT: How did you produce *El pacto de Adriana?*[6]

Lissette Orozco (LO): Very slowly. It took me five years; you can see me in the film going through life stages. In 2011, I applied for production support from the state film fund but didn't get it. I reapplied but to no avail. During my pitch, they asked if I wanted to make this film to clear my aunt's image. So, I had to complete the film through crowdfunding and with non-Chilean funding, for example, from the Tribeca Film Festival. Only after being nominated for an award at the Berlin Film Festival did I receive Chilean state funding to complete the postproduction.

AT: How did you approach the script?

LO: I never imagined my film as a large, high-end production. Its strength is a well-developed script with a strong dramatic structure. Describing it at first as a film about my aunt, I realized that it wasn't she but I who was in conflict with her past. Hence, I became the central character. As is

---

[6]   Conversation conducted via Skype on 27 October, 2017. I videoed Orozco's responses in Spanish and then transcribed, translated into English, and edited them. Orozco reviewed earlier drafts and approved the final version of the interview. I thank her for her interest and support and for providing me with photographs, media materials, and access to her film.

common in documentary filmmaking, I constantly rewrote the script while events unfolded. My first draft outlined ideal events and potential directions. In the first scene of that draft, I arrive in Australia, call at my aunt's door, and then we talk in her flat. Yet, I never went to Australia. I knew that some of these ideal events were highly unlikely; for example, a scene where my aunt turns herself in to the police. I drafted that script to get a development grant, which I then used to procure Chilean filmmaker Iván Osnovikoff's assistance. This made the script more real, but the film's structure was only completed in the editing.

AT: Was the film difficult to direct?

LO: Although this wasn't my first directorial experience, it was my first feature-length film. Because the production lasted years, I had to become acquainted with changing crew members many times. The use of multiple formats was new to me, including my dad's family video and footage of my aunt filming herself. I also use video that I shot of my conversations with my aunt, my grandmother, and my great-grandmother. The intimacy in these scenes would have been impossible had there been someone else doing camera or sound. And I include research video, which I wasn't thinking of using in the film at first. There is also professionally shot video of interviews and public events, such as the homage to Pinochet and the commemoration of the fortieth anniversary of the coup in 2013, where I had camera operators and a sound recordist with me. On these shoots, I was in front of the camera and had a second camera farther away documenting the filmmaking process.

AT: How would you describe your film's style?

LO: This film basically narrates my coming to terms with my aunt's case. So, there is a meta-textual level that runs through the narrative, for example, when I reflect in voice-over about the significance of a scene both for the film and for me. These structural elements and the combined use of materials from multiple sources give the film a characteristic collage-like style that resembles a video journal. In fact, initially I was just trying to keep a video record of my experiences.

AT: When did you decide to make a full documentary?

LO: Officially, I started *El pacto de Adriana* the first time I spoke publicly about it in 2011. But without realizing it, I had started much earlier when I decided to keep the paper with the news of my aunt's arrest in 2007. From then on, I instinctively kept saving information about her case. Around 2009, I was drafting a fiction film script based on the case of Rodrigo Anfruns, a six-year-old child abducted and murdered in Santiago in 1979, and my mum said to me: "Why don't you ask your Aunt Chany, she worked for DINA and may know something". I approached her hesitantly, but she didn't have any problem with giving me a video interview, which was the first I did with my aunt. By the time of my second interview, sometime before her escape from Chile in 2011, I knew I was making a documentary related to her case.

AT: How did your aunt respond to the documentary idea?

LO: Given that in 2011 I was close to finishing my Master's, I knew very well that I had to get my aunt to sign a clearance form immediately. I told her I wanted to make a documentary connected to her case, but that the film would focus on me rather than her; on what it meant for me to find out about her past. She said: "OK, make it about you, and I will demonstrate to you that I'm right". I agreed, and she signed the form.

AT: What was it like for you to discover your aunt's past as a DINA agent?

LO: It's been a daunting experience, and I'm still working through it. If my mum had been the one implicated, I wouldn't have made this film. But with Aunt Chany, I had a relationship at a distance. She would visit from Australia occasionally and would stay with us for a month, with the whole family revolving around her. And then she would leave. As an aunt, she was always caring, but she'd always been just an idealized character for me. I saw in her an imposing female figure who told the men in my conservative family right from wrong. But I knew little about her. If someone had asked me about her character, I would not have been able to say much. By making the film, and then having her around when she was on parole, I started to know what she was really like, for example, her authoritarian demeanor. I remember times when I'd be in the shower, and suddenly she'd turned off the hot water since, according to her, "five minutes in the shower was enough". I was shocked that she would intrude in my life like that. I realized she was a tough, domineering woman, but she was my aunt, and I respected her. After she fled Chile, we continued to interact via phone and internet. I sent her a video camera to Australia for her to keep a video diary for the film. I only asked her to describe to me whatever she felt like recording from her everyday life. But eventually, our communication started to break down. She became less open to me because I would always argue with her. You can see in the film how she grows suspicious of me because I'm no longer believing her denials. I found it quite impossible to accept her claim that she didn't know that DINA was torturing prisoners when she was a member. We'd have these clashing conversations that made my head spin. Sometimes, she would boldly justify the use of torture, and I would say to her: "That is awfully inhuman". During the production of the film, I started to discover that she wasn't the person I thought she was, that she had a dreadfully dark side. But then I'd get home and find a message from her saying: "Hello, dear, how are you? I love you". I didn't know what to do. I was constantly struggling with a desire to believe her. Sometimes, I felt like abandoning the project or wondered whether I could turn it into a fiction to avoid the conflict. I think I got started on this in quite a naïve way, and only now, after speaking publicly about it all year, I'm starting to see the dimension of what I did. One day, she sent me all the videos she'd made. What she did was to stage apparently candid scenes of her life in Australia, which were, however, related to her case. For example, she filmed herself crying while watching a television program about her case or talking with me on the phone or Skype but without telling me that she was filming. I was so impressed by the material she sent me that in the end, it became a good portion of the film. Possibly, this is the reason why she said that I used and betrayed her.

AT: Do you feel that you betrayed her?

LO: I sent my aunt a video camera to give her the opportunity to tell her side of the story. I did my best to be fair to her in the film. I showed what she recorded without adding commentary, and I never passed judgment on her. I also did everything she told me. In the film, she says: "Go and talk to such and such, show them this picture, ask them about this or that". I came to understand much later that she was doing all this to build her alibi. But her story collapses on camera because none of her former colleagues is willing to confirm her statements. They say they don't remember. Some even tell her that she's lying. In her footage, she contradicts herself, pressures me to threaten people, and tries emotional blackmail on me. I became aware of her manipulations only when I was editing the film. I realized I had to make a decision in order to finish it. I had to make myself responsible for what she was telling me and for so much evidence against her. So, if I've betrayed my own family, it's because I've made public their dark secret, and if I betrayed my aunt, it's because I didn't use my film to clear her image, as she expected me to do. On the other hand, I've been just toward many people whose lives were injured by her actions as a member of DINA. I do not make films just for my family. If I had used my documentary to clear my aunt's image, I would have rescinded my right to call myself a filmmaker. With her voluntary participation in the film, my aunt had the opportunity to reclaim her humanity. I don't judge the nineteen-year-old Adriana Rivas. I actually see her as another victim of that system. She could have said: "I was young when I got involved with DINA. They convinced me that I was on the right side, that we were fighting terrorists. But we were wrong to do what we did". But I cannot accept that now, in her sixties, she should continue to justify their actions and show pride for her time with DINA.

AT: How did others in your family react?

LO: The film was like a bomb that deeply fractured my extended family. To finish it, I had to struggle against most of my family, since they tried to stop me for over five years. My mum, of course, supports me. My cousins are also with me wholeheartedly. We are from a generation born in democracy and are not afraid of speaking out. My dad and his sisters, on the other hand, would say to me: "You are so talented, you could make a film about any other topic. Why do you want to make trouble for yourself?" And my right-wing uncles on my aunt's side would say threatening things like: "I hope you are not making a communist film! You are not going to fuck Chany up, are you?" I'd say to them: "I'll show whatever I find out". They'd argue: "You don't have any right to talk about things of which you know nothing, things that happened before you were even born!" Somehow, they made me feel like I was intruding into something with which I had nothing to do. Why can I not speak about the past, especially if it has directly affected me? These uncles won't speak to me now, and they've even threatened me with legal action. This is why their faces had to be blurred in the film. My family prefers to live in a constant state of amnesia, and I will never endorse that. In fact, I feel that my family's fissure has been more healing than damaging for me. In any case, I accept that I can easily say all this now that I'm travelling and constantly talking about the film. But I'm also processing all this stuff and I'm not totally sure what I may feel in the future. Regardless, I'm also constantly being reassured that my film contributes to the memory process in Chile.

AT: How has the public responded?

LO: Although *El pacto de Adriana* may not be a choice for the majority of Chileans who go to the cinema seeking entertainment, my film is today in its fourth week screening in commercial cinemas in Chile. This is something very unusual for a Chilean film in this country, even more rare if it's a documentary, and further still if it's about the dictatorship. So, this is a fantastic outcome and it's very encouraging to know that more people are becoming interested. There have been some very reassuring moments too. For example, after a screening in Valparaiso, one woman said: "I'm the daughter of one of the dictatorship's disappeared. Do you mind if I come up there and give you a hug?" It's also encouraging to show my film in countries where Chilean exiles live, to know that they are touched by it and to hear their own experiences. The film has been quite revelatory to many young Chileans as well, who've told me that the dictatorship topic cannot be brought up within their own families. Somebody told me that their grandfather was in the military during the dictatorship but nobody in the family wanted to speak about it. I recently received an email from a woman telling me that she and her family had not seen my film yet but that it depended on what they saw whether they would talk to her mother-in-law again. I asked who her mother-in-law was, and she happened to be one of my aunt's former DINA colleagues. I can only take responsibility for my own family's fracture. I don't know how many more Chilean families are going to implode as a result of my film. It has been screening all year nationally and internationally and has received many awards, including the Peace Award at the Berlin Film Festival, one of the world's top film events. It was also nominated for the Phoenix Awards, where it will be competing against the work of Latin American film masters. Regardless of the outcome, I feel I'm a winner already! I think the reason why this modest film is doing so well is that it appeals to audiences everywhere. It elicits strong responses because in spite of the story's Chilean context, the theme of digging out family secrets is universal . . . and stories about dictatorships are also universal.

AT: How do you think your film contributes to the memory process in Chile?

LO: My film shows that the only way not to distort or repeat history is to remember it. That half of Chileans prefer to live in a kind of amnesia is in itself one of this nation's greatest wounds. I grew up in a right-wing family where I often heard them say: "Why do these people insist on stirring up the past? Why do they need to be constantly remembering painful things that are better left to rest? When will they turn the page over so that we can live in a better country?" But, really, would you ever stop looking for and remembering a missing loved one? You can see in my film that today's Chile is still a nation deeply divided but also that it is not necessary that everybody agrees with everybody else for the truth to come out. I can empathize much more now with the victims, and I finally understood what they mean by "neither forgetting nor forgiving". It is simply not possible to forget or forgive the perverse acts that were committed under the pretense of intelligence work. Besides, survivors are not expecting anyone to ask them for forgiveness. What they seek is the bare truth about what happened to their relatives. They want to know where they can leave a flower in memory of their disappeared. Toward the end of *El pacto de Adriana*, I say that I see my film as my individual contribution to the memory process in Chile, that I hope it may motivate those who have information to come out and help to complete Chile's memory jigsaw puzzle. I also hope it will motivate others to talk and reflect about things that have been kept hidden for too long, and confront those who prefer to live in a state of amnesia.

5. Conclusions

Chilean political documentarians have investigated, uncovered, and depicted the dictatorial state's crimes while offering testimonial space to survivors and have also interrogated the perspectives of the dictatorship's supporter, collaborator, and perpetrator while wrestling with an open dialectic of confrontational and reconciliatory gestures, oscillating between critical confrontation and the desire for reconciliation, sometimes unyieldingly resorting to public denunciation and rupture within their own families. In the above conversations with three second-generation directors of post-dictatorship Chilean documentaries—Adrian Goycoolea's ¡*Viva Chile Mierda!* (2014), Andrés Lübbert's *El color del camaleón* (2017), and Lissette Orozco's *El pacto de Adriana* (2017)—this article has evidenced some of the complexities involved in the interrogation of the perspective of the dictatorship's collaborator. The article's interviews suggest that this is an especially challenging process when this scrutiny is performed by a personal narrator-director who is a member of the family of a willing or forced collaborator or a direct relative of those who have personally engaged with a collaborator. In the text of the above conversations, the reader can perceive how these young directors grapple with the shifting, problematic, and interrelated dynamics of confrontation and reconciliation, ultimately contributing with their nuanced narrations to an agonistic process of social reconciliation while departing in greater or lesser measure from the official restorative narrative of the Chilean democratic state's post-dictatorship monumental memory discourse.

Conflicts of Interest: The author declares no conflicts of interest.

References

Goycoolea, Adrian. 2014. ¡*Viva Chile Mierda! [Long Live Chile, Damn It!]*. Directed by Adrian Goycoolea. Brighton: Adrian Goycoolea.

Lübbert, Andrés. 2017. *El color del camaleón [The Color of the Chameleon]*. Directed by Andrés Lübbert. Cologne: 3boxmedia.

Lübbert, Andrés. 2016. *Dying for Life*. Directed by Andrés Lübbert. Antwerp: Andrés Lübbert.

Lübbert, Andrés. 2014. *Fistful of Memories*. Directed by Andrés Lübbert. Antwerp: Andrés Lübbert.

Lübbert, Andrés. 2009. *The Reality*. Directed by Andrés Lübbert. Antwerp: Andrés Lübbert.

Said, Marcela, and Jean de Certau. 2011. *El mocito [The Young Butler]*. Directed by Marcela Said, and Jean de Certau. Santiago: Centro Arte Alameda/Gitano Films.

Orozco, Lissette. 2017. *El pacto de Adriana [Adriana's Pact]*. Directed by Lissette Orozco. Buenos Aires: Meikincine.

Orozco, Lissette. 2014. *Subsuelo [Underground]*. Directed by Lissette Orozco. Bogotá: Lissette Orozco.

Orozco, Lissette. 2014. *Vorágine [Vortex]*. Directed by Lissette Orozco. Bogotá: Lissette Orozco.

Orozco, Lissette. 2010. *El día ideal [The Ideal Day]*. Directed by Lissette Orozco. Bogotá: Lissette Orozco.

Castillo, Carmen, and Guy Girard. 1994. *La Flaca Alejandra [Skinny Alexandra]*. Directed by Carmen Castillo, and Guy Girard. Paris: Institut National de l'Audiovisuel (INA).

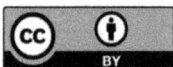

humanities

MDPI

Article

What Lies in the Gutter of a Traumatic Past: *Infancia clandestina* [*Clandestine Childhood*], Animated Comics, and the Representation of Violence

María Ghiggia

Independent Researcher, La Crosse, WI 54601, USA; ghiggia.maria@gmail.com

Received: 11 December 2017; Accepted: 1 March 2018; Published: 6 March 2018

Abstract: This essay focuses on the animated comics in the representation of violence in Benjamín Ávila's *Infancia clandestina* [*Clandestine Childhood*] (2011), a cinematic narrative of the seventies in Argentina. Drawing from animation and comic studies and adopting a formalist approach, the following analysis proposes ways in which the remediation of comics in the film underscores traumatic aspects of state terror and revolutionary violence and the problematic intergenerational transmission of memory of the 1970s–1980s militancy. Specifically, I comment on how the switch from photographic film to the animated frames draws attention to the blank space between the frames and thereby hints at the traumatic in what is left out, repressed, or silenced. While the gaps resist the forward motion of closure, paradoxically they allow for the suture of the frames/fragments in a postmemorial narrative, although not without a trace of the traumatic. Finally, extending the concept of the gutter as a liminal space, I analyze the connection between the animated scenes representing violence and the testimonial and documentary elements placed in the closing titles, a connection that asserts the autobiographical component of the film and enacts the conflictive character of intergenerational memory.

Keywords: comics; violence; Argentine film; children of the disappeared

It is a rainy night in 1975 in Argentina. A young couple and their seven-year-old child get off a bus and hastily walk back to their home on a quiet street in a city neighborhood. As the mother rushes to unlock the door, the father spots a quickly approaching car. An arm protrudes from the car and starts shooting. Having been warned by her husband, the woman pushes the child down to the sidewalk. At this moment, the live-action film abruptly switches into an animated sequence that alternates between frames of the adults shooting back at the car and close-ups of the terrified child. Eventually, the car drives away, and the shooting dies out. The last frame in the animated sequence is a still shot taken from above, with the camera circling around. It shows the child lying with his face down on the sidewalk and the parents crouching beside him. A yellow thread emerging from below the child's waist meets a red thread pouring out of the father's knee. So begins *Infancia Clandestina* [*Clandestine Childhood*] (2011), a film that adopts the point of view of a child named Juan to tell the story of the son of revolutionary militants in the 1970s in Argentina. In 1979, after spending four years in exile, the boy and his baby sister return to the country with their parents, who, along with other militants, launch a counteroffensive against the repressive military junta that ruled Argentina between 1976 and 1983.

The shootout described above is one of three scenes in the film in which the most violent, most traumatizing moments in Juan's story are represented through a hybrid of animation and comics. In her analysis of Spiegelman's *Maus*, Marianne Hirsch interprets the "bleeding" in Art Spiegelman's subtitle of *Maus I* ("My father bleeds history") as a metaphor for "loss" in the intergenerational transmission of traumatic events and collective tragedies (Hirsch 2012, p. 34). As has been noted, in the last frame of the first sequence of animated comics in *Infancia clandestina* the red (blood) meeting yellow (urine) can be interpreted as "a similar metaphor" for "this [other] traumatic intergenerational legacy" in this cinematic narrative by a son of militants committed to armed struggle in the sixties and seventies in Argentina (Maguire 2017, p. 138). Taking a closer look at this last frame, one can observe that the yellow thread of urine, symbolizing fear, meets blood red *in the space between the sidewalk tiles.* Blood oozing from the father's wound, a word etymologically associated with trauma, runs *in between the tiles.* That liminal space resembles a gutter in comics, the blank space between panels. I contend that the last frame in the opening scene of *Infancia clandestina* offers a self-reflexive commentary on its intermediality, drawing attention to the gutter and underscoring how the remediation of comics hints at the traumatic character of violence in the seventies in Argentina within intergenerational memory.[1]

The gutter has been theorized in comics studies in connection to trauma as the space of the Real (Ault 2000; Chute 2016), "not the actual space of non-representation" but "instead the space that *figures* some representation or narrative action left out" (Chase 2012, p. 113). Steve McCloud defines the gutter as the space in which "closure" takes place, the process by which readers fill in the gaps, imagining the transitions between two frames (McCloud 2008, p. 63). Referencing Eisenstein's discussion of montage, Gregory Chase indicates a parallel between comics and film based on both these media's dependence "on closure through a mechanism of non-representation (for film; the cut; for comics, the gutter) through repetition" (Chase 2012, p. 124). While McCloud does not problematize closure, other critics warn against the illusion of filling the void and highlight the persistence of a "residual trace" (Ault 2000, p. 126), a reminder of "the ever-present threat of the Real" (Chase 2012, p. 114). Likewise, while McCloud interprets closure as a forward motion, Chase points out the gutter's resistance to it (Chase 2012, p. 115).

Adopting a formalist approach to the animated comics in *Infancia clandestina*, this analysis illuminates the memory processes at work in the construction of this posttraumatic cinematic narrative. The switch from the photographic film to the animated comics calls attention to the gaps between the frames, and by doing this, it hints at the traumatic in what is left out, lost, repressed, or silenced in the violent scenes. The remediation of comics stages a resistance to the forward motion in the "jumpy" feel of the animated frames. Paradoxically, it is the stillness and the void of the gaps between the frames (the gutters) that enable the narrative in the film to move forward in attempting to suture the wounds from the past. If the animated frames can be interpreted as mediating personal, collective, and cultural memories of the violence in the 70s, the gaps between the frames resist closure and point to the traumatic as a residue or trace. This paradox resonates with Hirsch's characterization of postmemory as "an uneasy oscillation between continuity and rupture ... a structure of inter- and transgenerational return of traumatic knowledge and embodied experience" (Hirsch 2012, p. 6).

The incorporation of comics in *Infancia clandestina* could be seen against a background of cases of intermediality in other narratives that deal with the remembrance of collective tragedies and traumatic events. As intermedial representational technologies that combine text and images, print comics and graphic narratives have gained much popularity and recognition in recent decades, contributing to and benefitting from what W. J. T. Mitchell terms the "pictorial turn" (Heer and Worcester 2009, p. xi). Spiegelman's *Maus* is arguably the most globally renowned example of a work that uses comics to represent historical trauma. Despite initial objections, it has become clear that, as a recipient of a Pulitzer Prize, *Maus* set the stage for the production of graphic memoirs, graphic novels, and documentary

---

[1]   David Jay Bolter and Richard Grusin define remediation as "the formal logic by which new media refashion prior media forms" (Bolter and Grusin 1999, p. 273). The term not only applies to new technologies, however, but is broadly understood as "the mediation of remediation," a process in which "[m]edia are continually commenting on, reproducing, and replacing each other" (Bolter and Grusin 1999, p. 55).

comics.[2] The pictorial turn has extended its influence across national borders and cultures. As Chiara De Cesari and Ann Rigney point out, "globalized communication" allows for the circulation of "the modes and aesthetics of remembrance practiced around the globe and the discourses informing them" (De Cesari and Rigney 2014, p. 12).

The emergence of comics and graphic art as media to interrogate the traumatic past of political violence and state terror in the Southern Cone can be partly attributed to these global trends.[3] Jorge Catalá Carrasco, Paulo Drinot, and James Scorer attribute the suitability of comics as "mediums or technologies of memory" to their formal features which have led to "the development of a series of visual techniques that enable the rendering of memory (or memories) in distinct and often sophisticated ways" (Catalá Carrasco et al. 2017, p. 5). Besides *Infancia clandestina*, other postdictatorship works that employ comics in approaching traumatic aspects of the past are *Historietas por la identidad* [Comics for Identity][4], *Zombies en la Moneda* [Zombies in La Moneda] (2009), Roberto Santullo and Matías Bergara's *Acto de guerra* [Act of War] (2010)[5], and Carlos Trillo and Lucas Varela's *La herencia del coronel* [The Colonel's Legacy] (2010). Catalá Carrasco, Drinot, and Scorer point out two examples of transmediality in postdictatorship Argentina that instantiate comics "as sites of memory beyond the page" (Catalá Carrasco et al. 2017, p. 16). Both works remediate motifs, characters, and scenes from comics by Héctor G. Oesterheld, a major figure in Argentine and Latin American comics who was disappeared by the military junta in 1978.[6] The first is Félix Saborido's "¿DONDE ESTA OESTERHELD?" ['Where is Oesterheld?'], a poster that shows a crowd composed of Oesterheld's characters with a banner denouncing the artist's disappearance. The other work, by artist Lucila Quieto, combines scenes from Oesterheld's comics series *Sargento Kirk* with photographs of the 1969 uprising in Córdoba.

Discussions on intermediality in postdictatorship narratives in South America concern themselves with the increasing mass-media dissemination of images of collective tragedies, the effect of that dissemination on the remembrance of these traumatic events, and more specifically a "deterritorialization" of images (Andermann 2012; King 2013). Jens Andermann focuses on "the tension between static photographic image and the moving cinematic image" in posttraumatic autobiographical and autofictional documentaries in Argentina (Andermann 2012, p. 178). Andermann sees a productive form of deterritorialization in "the cinematic chronotope" that "mobilizes and itinerates a melancholy caught up in monumental immobility" (Andermann 2012, p. 178). In his analysis of literary narratives in postdictatorship Brazil, Edward King points out the "tensions between text and image," which reveal an uneasiness with the growing "mediation of memory" and "the blurring of the boundaries between individual and collective memory, key processes" in Hirsch's postmemory and Alison Landsberg's prosthetic memory (King 2013, p. 88). Hirsch invests "photographic images," especially family photographs, with a form of "affective" or "affiliative" memory that "re-embod[ies]" the past and "address[es] the spectator's own bodily memory"

---

[2]   Other often cited graphic works are Marjane Satrapi's *Persepolis: The Story of a Childhood* (2000–2003) and Joe Sacco's comics journalism, including *Palestine* (1996) and *Footnotes in Gaza* (2009).

[3]   In Argentina, a major incentive for the production of graphic narratives examining aspects that had been previously silenced was a shift in human rights discourses and memory politics after the economic and political crisis of 2001 (Fernández 2016, pp. 193–94).

[4]   *Historietas por la identidad* is a series of comic strips by various artists based on the testimonies of siblings of individuals who were taken as infants from their biological mothers and given away by the military during the Argentine 1976–1983 dictatorship. Andy Riva, who created the animated comics for *Infancia clandestina*, collaborated in this project sponsored by the human rights organization Abuelas de Plaza de Mayo [Grandmothers of Plaza de Mayo]. See (Asociación de Abuelas de Plaza de Mayo and Biblioteca Nacional 2015).

[5]   *Acto de guerra*, a collection of stories based on testimonies of armed struggle in Uruguay, presents a more critical outlook on revolutionary organizations than the Argentine film by addressing controversial issues such as members who acted as informants to the military and were seen as traitors.

[6]   Héctor G. Oesterheld was a member of Montoneros, as were his four daughters, also victims of the 1976–1983 dictatorship's brutal repression. His most famous character, "El Eternauta,"the eponymous character from the comics series of the same name, became a symbol of resistance.

(Hirsch 2012, pp. 38–39). King, on the other hand, argues for a different form of affect in the deterritorialization of images in image-texts (graphic narratives) that responds to "a desire to explore affective unbindings and reconfigurations rather than" "re-individualization" (King 2013, p. 97).

The focus of the current article is the effect of the interaction between the formal features of comics and film on the production of meaning in the remembrance of state terror and political violence in Argentina. As in Andermann's study, the contrast between stillness and motion plays an essential role in the remediation of comics in *Infancia clandestina*. However, rather than monumentalization, the stillness in the gaps between the animated frames points to the traumatic as something that has been left out or silenced in this narrative about the recent past in Argentina. In part, it could be argued that, as a distancing device, the animated comics may engage viewers by virtue of a form of affect understood as "intensity" that differs from emotion and "affective memory" (King 2013, p. 89). Yet this film still relies on "affective memory" in its inclusion of autobiographical family photographs as "structures" of postmemory (Hirsch 2012, p. 33).

Infancia clandestina is the work of director Benjamín Ávila, whose mother was a disappeared member of Montoneros, a revolutionary organization that originated as the left-leaning faction of *peronismo* [Peronism], a political movement founded by Argentine president Juan Domingo Perón. In composing the story, the director (born 1972) drew from his childhood experience. He is between the generation of his militant mother and that of children who were too young to remember the 1970s or were born after the dictatorship. Like the characters in the film, after some years in exile in Brazil, Mexico, and Cuba, Ávila returned to Argentina with his mother and her Montonero militant partner; both were engaged in the counteroffensive against the military regime (Kairuz 2012). Juan's birthday party, his grandmother's secret and unexpected visit, and the child's close and loving relationship with his parents were all part of Ávila's experience (*Revista Cabal* 2012). Just as with the child protagonist, as the son of a guerrilla in the Argentina of 1979, Ávila had to be careful about not giving away his real identity and endangering his family and himself.

On the other hand, *Infancia clandestina* is not strictly autobiographical. Whereas Ávila was seven years old when he returned to Argentina, the child character in the film is twelve. Neither the "real" name (Juan, after Juan Domingo Perón) nor the alternate name the parents select for their child to use as part of his underground identity (Ernesto, after Ernesto "Che" Guevara) matches the director's name. As has been pointed out, the film's "representational regime" is fictional, "with actors playing all roles and the action firmly set in the historical past of 1979" (Thomas 2015, p. 237). The director was interested in creating a story that was not centered on himself. In an interview he states that he needed to gain distance, that "quería correr[se] del centro" ['he wanted to step aside'], an expression that implies the displacement or decentering of the self that is enacted in the story by the child's dual identity (Kairuz 2012). While Juan's life with his militant family seems closer to Ávila's own clandestine childhood, Juan's alternate identity as Ernesto provides an outlet for the creative impulse. The coming-of-age archetype with its conventions serves as the model to invent situations and characters such as María, Ernesto's school friend and his first love. The narrative moves between these two stories with the child struggling to keep his two worlds separate and to balance the risks of his childhood as the son of revolutionaries under the military regime with his role as a somewhat ordinary school boy who falls for a friend's sister (María). Ávila intended this parallel story to be a way of emphasizing the domestic and ordinary despite the violence: "Because of the violence in Juan's world, the outside world had to have the same weight just to push Juan to the side" (*Director Talk* 2013).

The presence of testimonial and documentary elements at the end of the film, however, suggests an unwillingness to relinquish the autobiographical dimension completely. Both the dedication to Ávila's mother and the family photographs in the closing titles encourage the spectator to reconsider the story in light of the autobiographical connection. The photographs allow for the possibility of analyzing the film in terms of memory by pointing to the director's childhood and introducing "a trace of the present-ness into the film (as they are now objects of memory examined from a present vantage point)" (Thomas 2015, p. 241). As a work in which personal, cultural, and collective memories of the seventies' militancy intersect, the film draws attention to its representational and aesthetic choices, particularly regarding the portrayal of violence.[7] To this day, revolutionary violence remains one of the most controversial issues about the seventies in Argentina, and it constitutes an arena of contestation in the construction of memories of this period. The revision of political violence in the 1970s demands an examination that avoids mystification or demonization of it. While still defending the convictions and commitment to social justice of their generation, some former militants denounce the militarization of organizations such as Montoneros and the irresponsibility of their leaders, abandonment of politics in favor of violence, and refusal to accept failure.[8] In the case of children of former militants, stances in regard to their parents' militancy are far from monolithic, with some being more overtly critical than others.

Whether *Infancia clandestina* is approached as primarily fictional or autobiographical has consequences for how the film in general and the animated scenes have been critically received. The animated scenes in Ávila's film have been used in support of arguments that revolve around two aspects of the film. Some critics focus on the construction of the child's viewpoint and the contribution of the animated frames as a way of foregrounding the "alterity" of the child's gaze in the representation of violence (Thomas 2015; Maguire 2017). The other aspect that has been discussed extensively is the representation of the guerrilla and revolutionary organizations in Argentina and the endorsement of an image of their militancy as heroic and idealistic (Aguilar 2013; Garibotto 2015).[9] While these readings acknowledge to various degrees the autobiographical and documentary elements, they downplay them in favor of a view of the film as a fictional account of the seventies in which the child is a symbolic figure whose conflict symbolizes the "central conflict within the militant groups of that period, namely the tension between the pleasures of everyday life and sacrifice to a form of militant action that could result in death" (Aguilar 2013, p. 22).[10]

These articles that direct their attention to the representation of militancy make a much-needed contribution to the study of *Infancia clandestina* by contextualizing the discussion within memory politics and within Argentine politics of the time. Placing the film in its local historical and political contexts elucidates aspects that are presented vaguely in this historically-based film, such as the adult characters' views toward the armed struggle within guerrilla organizations.[11] On the other hand, while recognizing the relevance of *Infancia clandestina* as a cultural artifact that contributes to local debates on the recent past and whose production benefited from the political agenda and cultural initiatives in the 2010s, it is necessary as well to consider the reception of the film in global contexts. *Infancia clandestina* was also meant to be watched by audiences outside Argentina and to represent the country in the competition for Best Foreign Film at the Academy Awards. Movie reviews in English gravitated toward the child protagonist, his emotions, and his struggle to negotiate the dangers of his life as the child of militants with his childhood as a schoolboy.[12]

Ávila's film has been discussed in relation to Luis Puenzo's *La historia oficial* [*The Official Story*] (1985), the Oscar-winning film in which the disappeared are represented as victims, an image that became the hegemonic memory of the 1980s with the return to democratic rule in the country and the human rights organizations' fight for justice against the crimes of the military regime. The emblematic theory of the "two demons" (the military junta and the guerrillas) put forward by the CONADEP's report *Nunca más* [Never again] further cemented the representation of the disappeared as victims by

---

[7] To prepare for their roles the adult actors consulted former Montonero members. See (Pérez Zabala 2012).
[8] See (Elgueta 2013).
[9] Gonzalo Aguilar stresses "the idyllic" in the representation of the guerrilla figure through the lens of the child (Aguilar 2013, p. 26). Victoria Garibotto discusses the "iconizing" of an "archaic" image of the militancy from the 1970s through the child's romanticizing gaze (2015).
[10] See (Garibotto 2015, p. 266).
[11] See (Aguilar 2013, pp. 23–25) for an excellent discussion of different perspectives on this topic as represented in *Infancia clandestina*, including the confrontation between Juan's mother (Charo/Cristina) and grandmother (Amalia).
[12] See (Young 2012; Dargisjan 2013).

characterizing the violence of the seventies as "excesses" in the confrontation between two forces.[13] Not until the 1990s, when discussions of the militancy of the disappeared began, did the figure of the militant emerge and gain more visibility. While this figure challenged the demonization of the revolutionary organizations, groups within human rights organizations promoted a view of the militants as heroic, idealistic youth. Discourses on militancy and heroism were also encouraged in the 2000s by the human rights policies adopted by administrations of Argentine presidents Néstor and Cristina Kirchner. Ávila's ideological alignment with these policies has been noted in the criticism of the film.[14] While the director's political sympathies may be a bias in the representation of left-wing militancy in the film, it should be observed that the reception of a work is not limited to authorial intentions. This seems important when analyzing the animated comics in *Infancia clandestina*.

Released in 2011, Ávila's film, unlike *La historia oficial*, is not mainly concerned with the denunciation of the crimes of the military regime but with the experience and memories of children whose parents were militants. The focus of the narrative is the child; it is the child's viewpoint the film adopts, for the most part, in relating the story.[15] Spectators sympathize with the child and his emotions. There are some scenes in the live-action film in which the child's gaze may contribute to an idealized and iconized image of the militancy.[16] In a festive gathering of the militants before a secret operation against the military, for example, we see Juan watch the young militants. His eyes convey a certain fascination in the way he looks at the militants, including his parents. Juan's reverie is heightened by his mother's singing of a song that celebrates the idealism of youth. However, it is more difficult to make this case when it comes to the animated frames in which Juan appears as a witness to or a victim of acts of violence in which his parents and his uncle engage with death squads. Adopting the child's perspective, these scenes encourage the viewer's empathy with his distress and fear, emotions that are encoded by the cartoon drawings in the style of anime. As Sarah Thomas argues, it is in the animated scenes portraying violent events where the film most strongly encourages character-viewer identification (Thomas 2015, p. 247).

The arguments in favor of seeing these violent animated frames as serving a purely "auratic" and "symbolic" purpose invoke a "non-indexical" quality of cartoons.[17] Gonzalo Aguilar argues that the symbolic representation "subsumes the trauma of violence and defeat" (Aguilar 2013, p. 24). While I agree that the film is vague on debates and ideological views of the guerrilla organizations and does not question them or address their failure, I focus on the child and the spectator's identification with him. Viewing the film from this perspective, I propose that the shift from the live-action film to the animated frames highlights rather than suppresses the traumatic. Without spectacularizing violence, the media hybridization draws attention to violence, framing it. Rather than placing the focus on the content of the animated frames, the sudden switch in representational devices stirs in the spectator the feeling that something is left out in the spaces between the frames. It ultimately encourages the spectator to interrogate issues related to violence beyond state repression and resistance, calling to mind complexities and ethical ambiguities. In a way, these scenes underscore the gray zones of a story that draws on personal and collective memories of militancy. The remediation of comics in the film as

---

13 CONADEP, Comisión Nacional sobre la Desaparición de Personas [National Commission on the Disappearance of Persons], was an Argentine organization commissioned by President Raúl Alfonsín to investigate the violation of human rights by the military regime during the 1976–1983 dictatorship.

14 (Aguilar 2013, p. 19; Garibotto 2015, p. 268).

15 See Thomas for a detailed discussion of focalization and exceptions to this in the adoption of the child's gaze in the film.

16 Some images in the animated scenes could be interpreted as contributing to the "iconization" of 1970s militancy as heroic and/or sacrificial; these are two famous photographs of Ernesto "Che" Guevara, the Cuban revolutionary and guerrilla leader: the iconic photograph of Che with the beret taken by Alberto Korda in 1960 and the photograph of Che's corpse taken by Freddy Alborta in 1967. However, despite the symbolic character these images have acquired in cultural remembrance, overlapped with cartoons representing tragic events in the child's life, they stress the consequences of violence for the lives of ordinary people, including children.

17 Garibotto takes the term "auratic" from Walter Benjamin to characterize the child's gaze in the contemplation of the militants in the film (Garibotto 2015, p. 264). For a different view on comics as "indexical," see (Chute 2016, p. 21).

an aesthetics of remembrance points to the most traumatic aspects of this experience while it eludes any direct criticism not only of the 1970s militancy and revolutionary violence but also of the militants in their role as parents. In sum, the animated scenes highlight the complexity of personal, collective, and cultural remembrance, especially in cases of traumatic experiences.

In *Infancia clandestina*, Ávila uses multiple mediations in telling the story of his clandestine childhood: photographic or live-action film, animation in a style between motion comics or animation comics and anime (Japanese-style animation), graphic art in the form of drawings simulating photographs, and an animated segment that emulates a hand-drawn video featuring child-like drawings. These mediations represent distinct instances of graphic art and visual media that play different roles in the film. What sets apart the animated frames on which I focus here is the way the film remediates the conventions and aesthetics of comics in representing violent events in Juan's story. In all three scenes there is a sudden, unexpected shift from the photographic film to animation that occurs in the most dramatic moments and renders the child paralyzed with fear.

The first sequence of animated scenes is a shootout, as described previously, in which the boy's parents are attacked by members of a death squad. The text superimposed over the last frame provides a chronology that starts in 1974 with Perón's death and the persecution of militants by death squads[18]; it continues with the military coup in 1976 and the beginning of state terror and ends in 1979 with the Montoneros's return from exile to launch the Counteroffensive against the military junta. This first scene is set in 1975.

The second animated sequence is part of a nightmare that Juan has after learning that his beloved Uncle Beto has died. Juan's dream, which begins with live-action film, recreates in part what his father told him about his uncle's passing. Juan walks into a room in the house and finds his uncle sitting in a chair, smoking. They start a conversation that references a previous talk, a sort of initiation ritual in which Uncle Beto shares with his nephew his secrets on how to "deal" with girls. The photographic film shifts into animation just after they are ambushed by men in uniform and Uncle Beto pushes Juan down to protect him. What follows is a recreation of Juan's father's account of Uncle Beto's death. As Juan gazes in horror, Uncle Beto hugs a police officer and detonates a grenade as he pushes both of them into the back of his van. The scene that follows returns to the photographic film and shows Juan waking up in a state of shock with his mother trying to comfort him.

The third and last animated sequence is the most complex one, since it mixes images from different parts of the film, enacting a displacement of images that overlaps the present with the past. It appears after Juan learns from the news on television that his father has been killed. While the house where he lives with his family is raided by the death squads, Juan and his baby sister hide in the back room as his parents had instructed him. Once again, animation intervenes at the peak of the tension, in this case as the door is forced open by the death squad. At this moment, a flurry of images from previous parts of the film are remediated into animated frames and alternate with other frames that portray the death squads capturing Juan's mother and driving Juan away in a car.

The animated sequences in *Infancia clandestina* can be described as a hybrid between animation comics or motion comics and cell animation in the style of anime or limited animation. Motion comics is itself a hybrid that "combines formal attributes associated with comics and animation" such as still frames and panning or zooming, but, "the particular attributes remediated tend to differ on a case-by-case basis, making defining the medium's essential characteristics difficult" (Jeffries 2017, p. 203). Another feature is the expansion of individual panels into a full shot or remediation of single panels into single frames. Drew Morton points out formal affinities between motion comics and limited animation, which include the recycling of drawings, camera movements such as panning or zooming

---

[18] The groups attacking the militants in 1974 are identified in the film rather vaguely as "grupos parapoliciales" ['death squads']; there is no direct reference to the Alianza Anticomunista Argentina [Argentine Anticommunist Alliance], known as "Triple A," a far-right death squad created in 1973 and led by José López Rega, Minister of Social Welfare under Juan Perón until 1974 and then under Perón's wife and Vice-President, Estela Martínez de Perón, better known as Isabel Perón (1974–1976).

used to create the illusion of movement, and voiceover narration or dialogue between characters (Morton 2015, p. 351). In *Infancia clandestina*, rather than panning or zooming, animation relies more on a montage of still frames. Likewise, anime or Japanese animation features limited animation techniques, with lower cell count and plenty of still shots or images. Of particular interest to the aesthetics of the cartoons in the film is anime's emphasis on the characters' emotions as communicated through iconic facial expressions.

As I highlighted briefly above, the closing frame in the first scene in *Infancia clandestina* presents an image that condenses key points in my argument about the use of animation frames in the representation of violent scenes and its expressive potential to underscore traumatic aspects of violence in 1970s Argentina. The last frame in the dramatic shootout with blood running between the sidewalk tiles draws attention to the gutter, an element of comics that helps explain how comics and film convey motion and temporality differently: "Since comics consist entirely of static images and cinema features images that move, their respective relationships to time could hardly be more different" (Jeffries 2017, p. 18).

One concern when incorporating comics into film is how to remediate stasis as movement. The gutter, the space between the panels, is essential in understanding how time and motion are expressed spatially in comics as opposed to film in which the illusion of movement is produced with the projection of one frame after another. Bridging the temporal gaps and interpreting the relations between the panels is a process in which the comics reader plays an active role. This is what McCloud calls "closure" (McCloud 2008, p. 63). Therefore, it is incompleteness and rupture that define comics and give it a "staccato rhythm": "Comic panels fracture both time and space, offering a jagged, staccato rhythm of unconnected moments" (McCloud 2008, p. 67). In a similar way, Dru Jeffries illustrates the idea with an image he takes from David Carrier: "We construct a jumpy narrative, like a movie shown with the projector not quite in sync" (qtd. in (Jeffries 2017, p. 44)).

The animated frames representing violent events in *Infancia clandestina* draw attention to the gutter in the incorporation of comics into the film. It is the change of pace, an apparent contrast in the frame rate of the animated comics with that of the photographic film that produces an effect similar to that of a "jumpy narrative." In a regular speed film, images screened at a speed of twenty-four frames per second are perceived to be in continuous motion. This is what is known as "persistence of vision," the optical illusion by which the spectator interprets a sequence of still images as a continuous moving image. Thus, this speed renders the gaps between the frames as imperceptible. The switch from the photographic film to the animated frames emulates the incompleteness of comics; it hints at the gutter, the space between frames, which is still there but becomes invisible when each panel is remediated into a single frame in the film. By drawing attention to the gaps between the frames, the switch provokes an uneasy feeling that something has been left out in the montage. The absence/presence of the gutter in comics can be understood as "a mental negative space that is fueled with everything that isn't in the panels" (Marx 2007, p. 104).

Hillary Chute also understands the gutter in paradoxical terms, as a space between absence and presence, "both a space of stillness—a stoppage in the action, a gap—and a space of movement" (Chute 2016, p. 35). Chute's association of the gutter with stillness seems most relevant to my suggestions about the ways in which the change of pace in the violent scenes in *Infancia clandestina* makes the gutter stand out. This realization may lead to an exploration of the scenes in terms of what they hint at and what they leave out in the representation of violence. Chute goes on to propose that pace is crucial in a "work that approaches trauma, and seeks to approach histories of trauma" (Chute 2016, p. 37). According to Michael Levine, slowing down is what Spiegelman does in *Maus*. Interestingly, Levine chooses a cinematic metaphor to characterize Spiegelman's comics as a "slow-motion picture," an art between drawing and film, that sets in motion the static images at a slower pace than twenty-four frames per second, exposing the "interspaces," the gutters (Levine 2002, p. 320).

What links Chute's thoughts on the gutter even more closely to trauma, though, is the connection she proposes with the Lacanian Real: "To the extent that comics' formal proportions put into play what we might think of as the unresolvable interplay of elements of absence and presence, we could understand the gutter space of comics to suggest a psychic order outside of the realm of symbolization—and therefore, perhaps, a kind of Lacanian Real" (Chute 2016, p. 17). In an endnote, Chute expands on this: "Alan Sheridan describes Lacan's Real in language apposite to the gutter: 'the ineliminable residue of all articulation, the foreclosed element, which may be approached, but never grasped'" (Chute 2016, p. 272 n. 36). Donald Ault further explores the connection between the gutter and the Lacanian Real: "What is left over, the remainder in the blank space between the panels, performs the disruptive function of the real. There is nothing in this space, but it introduces discontinuities into the spaces of representation and allows the panels to assert themselves as fragments" (Ault 2000, p. 125). For Ault, the possibility of fixing or "suturing" this rupture through the symbolic and the imaginary in the process of reading is problematized by what Lacan calls the "gaze": "in our relation to things, in so far as this relation is constituted by way of vision, and ordered by the figures of representation, something slips, passes ... and is always to some degree eluded in it—that is what we call the gaze" (qtd. in Ault 126).

In *Infancia clandestina*, the switch from live-action film into the animated frames causes a disruption, intensified by the fact that it occurs *in media res*, at the highest peak of the dramatic tension in all three violent scenes, as I pointed out earlier. The second and third animated sequences contain discontinuities, expressed as the displacement of images that appear in other parts of the film. The last animated scene is probably the most complex and fragmentary. As mentioned before, the scene remediates, in the form of animation, some frames in the photographic film that appear earlier in the narrative, emulating the way flashbacks work. However, by suggesting that the change of pace or the "jumpiness" in these scenes might provoke in the viewer a feeling that something is missing, I do not point so much at these discontinuities within the sequences of animated frames. This feeling that something is lost could rather be interpreted as hinting at traumatic effects of the violence of the seventies in Argentina that cannot be accounted for because of the loss of life, the repressed, the forgotten, and the silenced. In pointing to the traumatic, the gutters alert us to its traces.

Just as in these violent scenes in which the representational medium underscores the gutter as a liminal or marginal space, the concept of the gutter can be used as an extended metaphor for the way *Infancia clandestina* is structured. In the organization of the film, the violent scenes fall into marginal spaces in the sense that, although they are not non-diegetic, they do not add much to the development of the narrative. This marginality, highlighted by the shift from the live-action film into animation, may be understood as an attempt on the part of the director to create a story that does not emphasize violence and horror as did earlier representations of state terror in the seventies. Violence is pushed to the side. In this sense, the violent scenes in themselves can be seen as gutters. Likewise, there are other elements in the film whose liminality is defined by their extradiegetic condition. As mentioned before, at the conclusion of the narrative, there is a dedication to the director's mother, Sara Zermoglio, who was disappeared in 1979. Immediately after this frame, a collection of Ávila's family photographs is screened alongside the closing titles. Echoing some scenes in the film that show Juan's family engaged in very "ordinary" and domestic situations despite the constant tension and fears of being found and captured by the military regime, these photographs portray Ávila's mother and Ávila himself as a child in similar scenarios. A few of the photographs show children playing at home and on the beach. One photograph features a birthday party, a memory that the director recreated in the story together with other autobiographical details. Photographs of Ávila's mother carrying a child (his youngest brother) bear a strong resemblance to frames in the film that show the actress playing Juan's mother carrying Juan's baby sister.

The family photographs, along with the dedication and other paratexts such as interviews with the director and movie reviews, underline the autobiographical connection. Even though the narrative is set entirely in 1979 and includes no framing device or adult character that links the present with the past, the paratexts create the possibility of interpreting the film in relation to postmemory (Thomas 2015, pp. 239–40). For Hirsch, photographs play a fundamental role in linking present and past, life and death, first- and second-generation memory: "Photographs in their enduring 'umbilical' connection to life are precisely the medium connecting first- and second-generation remembrance, memory and postmemory ... They affirm the past's existence and, in their flat two-dimensionality, they signal its unbridgeable distance" (Hirsch 2011, p. 23). Hirsch takes the image of the "umbilical cord" from Roland Barthes and his observations in *Camera Lucida* on photography as connected to life and death: "The photograph is literally an emanation of the referent. . . . A sort of umbilical cord links the body of the photographed thing to my gaze: light, though impalpable, is here a carnal medium, a skin I share with anyone who has been photographed" (Barthes [1980] 1981, pp. 80–81). The image of the "umbilical cord" and Hirsch's comment on its association with "life giving" and "maternity" (Hirsch 2011, p. 20) seem most appropriate and poignant when applied to Ávila's family photographs, particularly the photograph that portrays his mother pregnant with his youngest brother. Although Juan has a baby sister in the story, the abduction that occurs after the military ambushes the house at the end of the film coincides with the director's youngest brother's story.[19]

The inclusion of the dedication and the photographs in the closing titles makes a strong enough case for an interpretation of the film as autobiographical and as a work of memory. However, the film itself performs these connections in its aesthetic choices and its intermediality. It is important to notice that these photographs are placed against what appears as a cartoon wall; they are framed by an aesthetic of cartoons, which links them with the diegetic animated scenes representing violent, traumatizing events in Juan's story, including the forced disappearance of Juan's mother along with the baby. This is a concrete way in which the film can be said to stage the concept of postmemory, connecting Juan's story, based on Ávila's clandestine childhood, to Ávila's mother's story.

To re-evoke the closing frame in the first scene of the film, the connection between the photographs and the animated scenes representing violent events finds a metaphor in the image of the father's red blood meeting the child's yellow urine. As stated before, what underscores the traumatic character of the transmission of intergenerational memory of state terror and revolutionary violence is not just the bleeding, as in Spiegelman's tale of his father's survival, but rather the image of the blood running between the sidewalk tiles that resembles the gutter of comics. Both the photographs and the violent scenes can be seen to occupy a marginal space within the structure of the film. In this sense, they can both be understood as "gutters" in which the blood runs. As Thomas suggests, these photographs illustrate Barthes's *punctum* (Thomas 2015, p. 241). They are both reminders of life but, above all, of death and loss. In a similar way, the "jumpy" rhythm suggested by the pace in the screening of the animated comics insinuates that something is lost, left out in that representation. Rather than representing trauma, these scenes hint at the traumatic character of violence in this story that blends personal, collective, and cultural memories, by the son of a member of a guerrilla organization.

Conflicts of Interest: The author declares no conflict of interest.

References

Aguilar, Gonzalo. 2013. *Infancia clandestina* or the Will of Faith. *Journal of Romance Studies* 13: 17–31. [CrossRef]

Andermann, Jens. 2012. Expanded Fields: Postdictatorship and the Landscape. *Journal of Latin American Cultural Studies* 21: 165–87. [CrossRef]

Asociación de Abuelas de Plaza de Mayo, and Biblioteca Nacional. 2015. *Historietas por la identidad*. Edited by Judith Gociol. Ciudad Autónoma de Buenos Aires: Abuelas de Plaza de Mayo. (In Argentina)

Ault, Donald. 2000. 'Cutting Up' Again Part II: Lacan on Barks on Lacan. In *Analytical and Theoretical Approaches to Comics*. Edited by Anne Magnussen and Hans-Christian Christiansen. Copenhagen: Museum Tusculanum Press, pp. 123–39.

---

[19] Ávila's youngest brother was one of the babies kidnapped by the military and given to another family. His biological identity was revealed in 1984 thanks to Abuelas de Plaza de Mayo and their efforts to identify through DNA tests individuals who were taken from their mothers by the military during the 1976–1983 dictatorship.

Barthes, Roland. 1981. *Camera Lucida: Reflections on Photography*. Translated by Richard Howard. New York: Hill and Wang. First published 1980.

Bolter, Jay David, and Richard Grusin. 1999. *Remediation: Understanding New Media*. Cambridge: MIT Press.

Catalá Carrasco, Jorge L., Paulo Drinot, and James Scorer, eds. 2017. *Comics and Memory in Latin America*. Pittsburgh: University of Pittsburgh Press.

Chase, Gregory. 2012. 'In the Gutter': Comix Theory. *Studies in Comics* 3: 107–28.

Chute, Hillary L. 2016. *Disaster Drawn: Visual Witness, Comics, and Documentary Form*. Cambridge: Belknap Press of Harvard University Press.

Dargisjan, Manohla. 2013. Raised by Political Activists in a Dictatorship's Shadow. Available online: http://www.nytimes.com/2013/01/11/movies/clandestine-childhood-directed-by-benjamin-avila.html (accessed on 7 October 2017).

De Cesari, Chiara, and Ann Rigney. 2014. *Transnational Memory: Circulation, Articulation, Scales*. Berlin and Boston: Walter de Gruyter.

Director Talk. 2013. Clandestine Childhood/Benjamín Ávila. Available online: http://earthwize.org/wordpress/directortalk/2013/02/08/clandestine-childhoodbenjamin-avila/ (accessed on 7 October 2017).

Elgueta, Gloria y Claudia Marchant, ed. 2013. *Historia reciente y violencia política. Lucha Armada en la Argentina, la revista*. Santiago: Tiempo Robado.

Fernández, Laura Cristina. 2016. La historieta como relato de un trauma social en América Latina: Los casos *Historietas por la Identidad* (Argentina) y *Acto de Guerra* (Uruguay). *Miguel Hernández Communication Journal* 7: 191–215. [CrossRef]

Garibotto, Verónica Inés. 2015. Private Narratives and Infant Views: Iconizing 1970s Militancy in Contemporary Argentine Cinema. *Hispanic Research Journal* 16: 257–72. [CrossRef]

Heer, Jeet, and Kent Worcester, eds. 2009. *A Comics Studies Reader*. Jackson: University Press of Mississippi.

Hirsch, Marianne. 2011. Mourning and Postmemory. In *Graphic Subjects: Critical Essays on Autobiography and Graphic Novels*. Edited by Michael A. Chaney. Madison: The University of Wisconsin Press, pp. 17–44.

Hirsch, Marianne. 2012. *The Generation of Postmemory: Writing and Visual Culture after the Holocaust*. New York: Columbia University Press.

Infancia Clandestina [*Clandestine Childhood*]. 2011. Directed by Benjamín Ávila. Buenos Aires: Historias Cinematográficas and Habitación 1520 Producciones.

Jeffries, Dru. 2017. *Comic Book Film Style: Cinema at 24 Panels per Second*. Austin: University of Texas Press.

Kairuz, Mariano. 2012. Esto es lo Que Creo. Available online: https://www.pagina12.com.ar/diario/suplementos/radar/subnotas/8231-1802-2012-09-16.html (accessed on 7 September 2017).

King, Edward. 2013. Ekprhastic Anxiety and the Technological Mediation of Memory in Post-dictatorship Narratives from Brazil. *Journal of Romance Studies* 13: 88–98. [CrossRef]

Levine, Michael G. 2002. Necessary Stains: Spiegelman's *MAUS* and the Bleeding of History. *American Imago* 59: 317–41. [CrossRef]

Maguire, Geoffrey. 2017. *The Politics of Postmemory: Violence and Victimhood in Contemporary Argentine Culture*. Cham: Springer International Publishing.

Marx, Christy. 2007. *Writing for Animation, Comics, and Games*. Amsterdam and Boston: Focal Press.

McCloud, Scott. 2008. *Understanding Comics: The Invisible Art*. New York: HarperCollins Publishers.

Morton, Drew. 2015. The Unfortunates: Towards a History and Definition of the Motion Comic. *Journal of Graphic Novels and Comics* 6: 347–66. [CrossRef]

Pérez Zabala, Victoria. 2012. La Doble Vida de Juan. Available online: http://www.lanacion.com.ar/1508554-la-doble-vida-de-juan (accessed on 10 October 2017).

Revista Cabal. 2012. Entrevista a Benjamín Ávila, director de "Infancia clandestina". Available online: http://www.revistacabal.coop/actualidad/entrevista-benjamin-avila-director-de-infancia-clandestina (accessed on 7 September 2017).

Thomas, Sarah. 2015. Rupture and Reparation: Postmemory, the Child Seer and Graphic Violence in *Infancia clandestina* (Benjamín Ávila, 2012). *Studies in Spanish and Latin American Cinemas* 12: 235–54. [CrossRef]

Young, Neil. 2012. Clandestine Childhood: Cannes Review. Available online: http://www.hollywoodreporter.com/review/clandestine-childhood-cannes-review-327182 (accessed on 7 October 2017).

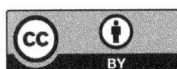

humanities

MDPI

Article

Between Grief and Grievance: Memories of Jews in France and the Klaus Barbie Trial

Michael G. Levine

German, Russian, East European Languages and Literatures, Rutgers University,
New Brunswick, NJ 08901, USA; mglevine@rci.rutgers.edu

Received: 21 September 2017; Accepted: 14 November 2017; Published: 21 November 2017

Abstract: Working between the Amos Gitai film *One Day You'll Understand* (2008) and the 1987 Klaus Barbie trial against which it is set, the article explores how the trial marked a decisive turning point in France's relationship to its wartime past. Of Barbie's hundreds of crimes, including murder, torture, rape, and deportation, only those of the gravest nature, 41 separate counts of crimes against humanity, were pursued in the French court in Lyon. Not only did the trial raise crucial juridical questions involving the status of victims and the definition of crimes against humanity but, extending into the private sphere, it became the occasion for citizens to address heretofore silenced aspects of their own family histories and conduct trials of a more personal nature. Whereas the law in general seeks to contain historical trauma and to translate it into legal-conscious terminology, it is often the trauma that takes over, transforming the trial into "another scene" (Freud) in which an unmastered past is unwittingly repeated and unconsciously acted out. Such failures of translation, far from being simply legal shortcomings, open a space between grief and grievance, one through which it is possible to explore both how family secrets are disowned from one generation to the next, and how deeply flawed legal proceedings such as the Barbie trial may "release accumulated social toxins" (Kaplan) and thereby expose unaddressed dimensions of French postwar (and -colonial) history.

Keywords: Klaus Barbie Trial; literary justice; crimes against humanity; testimony; traumatic flashback; French-Jewish memory; unconscious transmission; French resistance; filming of trials

> "It was not a story to pass on"
>
> Toni Morrison, *Beloved*

Much work has been done in recent years—primarily by legal scholars—on the vexed relationship between atrocity crimes and legal response. While deeply indebted to this work, I take as my own point of departure Shoshana Felman's path-breaking book *The Juridical Unconscious: Trials and Traumas of the Twentieth Century*, published in 2002, which stresses not only questions of jurisprudence but the unwitting repetition of historical trauma and the surprisingly unconscious dimension of the legal proceedings themselves. In the opening pages of her study, Felman describes this dynamic between trials and trauma in the following terms:

> The law tries to contain the trauma and to translate it into legal-conscious terminology, thus reducing its strange interruption. Uncannily, however, while the law strives to contain the trauma, it often is in fact the trauma that takes over and whose surreptitious logic in the end reclaims the trial . . . A pattern emerges in which the trial, while it tries to put an end to trauma, inadvertently performs an acting out of it. Unknowingly, the trial thus repeats the trauma, reenacts its structures . . . [L]ike society itself and despite its conscious frames and rational foundations, the law has quite conspicuously and remarkably its own structural (professional) unconscious (Felman 2002, p. 5).

For Felman, it is often the moments of collapse in juridical proceedings that are the most telling; for they give us surprising and otherwise unavailable access to the unconscious dimension of those trials. A case in point is her reading of the prosecution of Adolf Eichmann in which she focuses on a moment subsequently screened over and over on Israeli television like a traumatic flashback when the witness Yehiel Dinur—also known by his pen name, Ka-Tzetnik—suddenly falls silent and lapses into a coma on the witness stand. It is a moment when the witness feels himself torn between his two names and identities, between his place among the living and his vision of himself still among the dead and dying.

Elizabeth Rottenberg elaborates on the significance of such moments of collapse and failure, noting that what they "point to—insofar as they prove to be moments of legal and conceptual breakthrough—is a radical form of human grief". Although the Eichmann and Simpson trials examined by Felman are, in Rottenberg's words, both "concerned with the translation of grief into grievance, the jurisprudential *drama* of these cases is what finally succeeds in testifying to an abyss of mourning—an abyss to which a *literary* justice can, in the end, bear witness" (Rottenberg 2004, pp. 1102–3).

In what follows, I explore this relationship between grief and grievance and above all a certain *failure of translation* by which the two may be linked. I do so through an examination of Amos Gitai (2008) film *One Day You'll Understand* [*Plus tard, tu comprendras*], the 2005 memoir by Jérôme Clément on which it was based, and the 1987 Klaus Barbie trial against which it is set. While the complex relationship between the film and the memoir—not to mention the screenplay co-written by Clément and the book, *Maintenant je sais*, he would later write about the making of the film—deserve consideration in their own right, I wish to note at this point the surprising absence of any mention of the Barbie trial or even of Marcel Orphuls' documentary *Hotel Teminus: The Life and Times of Klaus Barbie* in Clément's original memoir. The absence is surprising given the works Clément, former director of the *Centre national de cinématographie* and founder of the influential television network ARTE, does discuss; these include Renais' *Night and Fog*, the Eichmann trial, Lanzmann's *Shoah*, Paxton's book on Vichy, Ophuls' *The Sorrow and the Pity*, Chirac's landmark 1995 address delivered on the anniversary of the Vel' d'Hiv' round up, the establishment in 1999 of a French Reparations Commission,[1] and the inauguration in 2005 of the Wall of Names at the *Mémorial de la Shoah* in Paris.

Only when writing the screenplay does Clément think to include the trial. As he recalls in his book about the making of the film, it was a visit in 2005 to the children's home in Izieu, the orphanage which Barbie had raided in 1944, rounding up the Jewish children he found there and sending them all to their death in Auschwitz, that first prompted Clément to reflect on the turning point in French postwar memory represented by the Barbie trial. As the trial judge, Pierre Truche, himself explained to Clément during his visit to Lyon:

> You have to understand what a decisive year 1987 was in terms of France's relation to its wartime past. For it was in that year that we first realized that Klaus Barbie was responsible not only for the assassination of Jean Moulin, hero of the Resistance, but also for the murder of Jewish children. What the Barbie trial brought to light was just how central the extermination of the Jews was to the Nazi regime. [Trans. mine] (Clément 2008, p. 280).

It was this new understanding of French history that prompted Clément to alter his memoir when adapting it for the screen. Whereas the memoir begins with the death of his mother in June 1996 and is conceived very much as a work of mourning, the film opens in May 1987 with the mother still very much alive and the Barbie trial in its eighth day. In the first scene in which the mother appears, the last part of which is carefully constructed as one long take, we see her become increasingly engrossed, almost against her will, in the Barbie trial being broadcast live on French television.

---

[1] La Commission pour l'indemnisation des victimes de spoliations intervenues du fait des législations antisémites en vigueur pendant l'Occupation (CIVS).

Recentering the original story in this way, the film draws attention to the act of witnessing—both the testimony given in the course of the trial and the witnessing of the trial by the French public. To make these two related forms of witnessing line up, the film takes certain liberties with the historical record, going so far as to incorporate archival footage of the trial first made available to the public only in 2007 into its narrative. Thus, unless one knows better, one has the impression in watching the film that contemporary audiences—including, of course, the protagonist's mother—had in fact been able to watch the trial proceedings live on French television in 1987.

Why would Gitai have resorted to this cinematic sleight of hand? Was it perhaps in order to draw attention to the broadcast politics of the times, a matter to which we will turn in a moment? Or was it simply a way of drawing attention to the central narrative conceit of the film? That conceit has to do with the interaction of private and public tribunals, with the implicit connection drawn in the film between trials conducted behind closed doors in many French homes at the time and the highly publicized, highly politicized trial of the notorious "Butcher of Lyon".

With regard to the broadcast politics of the Barbie trial, it should be noted that, as with Nuremberg and Eichmann, the proceedings were staged to serve the ends of both justice and didactic legality. Explaining this twofold agenda, the legal scholar, Lawrence Douglas, recalls how the French government described the Barbie prosecution as "a pedagogical trial," which in the words of Prime Minister Pierre Mauroy, would first "enable French justice to do its work, and second, ... honor the memory of that time of grieving and struggle by which France preserved her honor" (Douglas 2001, pp. 185–12). Douglas further notes that Minister of Communications Georges Filoud proposed broadcasting the trial live on French television, something without precedent in the annals of French broadcasting. Although Filoud's proposal was ultimately rejected, cameras *were* present in the Lyon courtroom—not to show the trial live on television but to record it for posterity, as the Parliament passed a law permitting the filming of important trials for historical purposes.[2]

As noted earlier, this archival footage was first made available in 2007, twenty years after the fact, and was used by Gitai in the scene in which the audience is first introduced to the protagonist's mother, played by the incomparable Jeanne Moreau (see Figure 1).

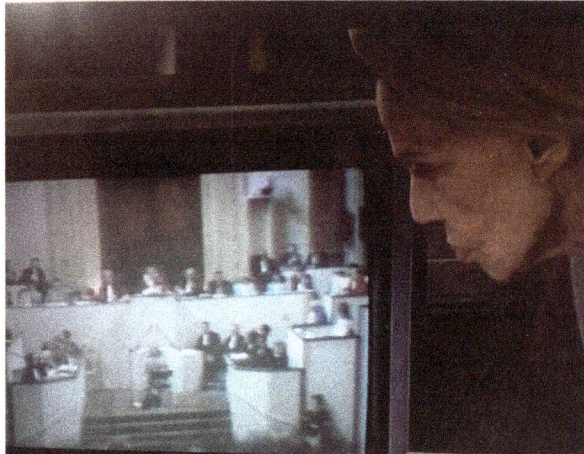

Figure 1. Testimony of Lea Katz.

---

[2]   See (Douglas 2001, pp. 185–86); see also (Rousso 1991, p. 201).

There is much to be said about this scene—about the way it gradually shifts from listening to viewing; about the point of the SS dagger and its strategic placement on the mantelpiece; about the relationship between the woman testifying in the trial and the one witnessing it from home; about the painful connection between words and wounds; and, of course, about the content of this particular testimonial excerpt. But because it is possible in the context of this article to focus only on static images rather than on entire cinematic scenes, I pass over these particular issues and consider instead the more general narrative and structural significance of the scene.

It is no exaggeration to say that the film remains stuck on this moment in the Barbie trial; for in the next scene, no longer set in the mother's home but instead in her son's office, the same testimony, that of Lea Katz, an eyewitness to the notorious roundup of Jews at the UGIF on 9 February 1943, is broadcast once again. This time, however, her testimony is heard on the radio instead of being seen on television (see Figure 2).

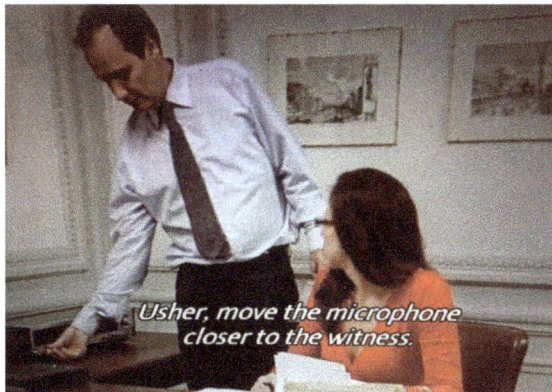

Figure 2. Radio Broadcast of Katz Testimony.

If the film moves in place at this particular instant, it does so for two related reasons: first, in order to underscore the significance of a certain moment *in* the trial and the apparent difficulty of getting beyond it; second, in order to stress the simultaneity of the two scenes of witnessing *of* the trial. Taking place at the same time, these scenes are effectively set in dialogue with each other. So not only do we see the mother and son, each following the trial in her or his own way, become increasingly implicated in it, but we also see the national wounds laid bare by the proceedings opening at the heart of the Bastien family, the father's side of which was Catholic, the mother's Jewish. As these wounds open, the scene of the trial itself shifts to the private sphere with the son now cast in the role of examining magistrate and the mother in the role of witness. Only now does the son seek to break the silence his mother had scrupulously maintained since the war about the deportation of her parents, the fate of their possessions, and her own relation to things Jewish.

As one might imagine, the trial conducted within the family has a very different tone from that of the official proceedings. Whereas in the latter, witnesses were subjected to intense questioning and often hostile cross-examination; judges were judged and the French legal system itself was put on trial by the radical defense attorney Jacques Vergès; and the very definition of crimes against humanity was altered for questionable political reasons having to do with the statute of limitations on war crimes, the claims of French Resistance groups, and the need of the government to shield itself from prosecution for crimes committed during the Algerian war; in the Bastien family, everything proceeds with utmost civility. Here, examiner and witness dance gently around each other. The son asks, the mother deflects, never exactly refusing to answer, just not now, *plus tard*.

As the title suggests, this is a film about time and understanding, about the ways in which the two never quite coincide. While comprehension seems to be what is promised, that promise is never exactly kept nor, for that matter, ever simply broken. Instead, it is kept only to the extent that it is kept open, kept in a state of abeyance. This is the side-stepping dance of deferral that mother and son, locked in an adversarial embrace, perform.

As the two turn around each other, asking and evading, the film itself turns in circles. For a long time, it doesn't seem to go anywhere and yet one feels the son's mounting frustration, his desire to probe held in check not just by his mother's resistance but by his own intuitive sense of just how far he can go. Needless to say, the more he restrains himself, the more intense his desire to know becomes. Indeed, the film slowly fills with this mounting tension. The air in the closed rooms of the family's Parisian apartments in fact becomes so thick, so saturated with lingering questions and evasive responses, that the characters are seen repeatedly opening windows and gasping for air.

As the tension both within and between these characters builds, the pace of the film increases, turning in ever tightening circles towards its center. That center is marked, not surprisingly, by another dance. Yet, before coming to it, Jérôme—or Victor as he is now called in Gitai's film—must himself perform a number of carefully choreographed preparatory steps involving a progression from writing to speaking to physical movement—as though the questions accumulating within him had the effect of mobilizing his energies and setting him literally in motion. Thus, in the first half of the film, we see him move successively from the papers scattered across his desk like the disordered family history he is trying desperately to sort out, to a series of verbal exchanges with his mother that go nowhere, to a car trip he takes with his wife and children to Salviac where he has arranged to meet with the mayor of the small southwestern French town in which his Jewish grandparents had been hidden.

The exchange between the two men starts slowly as the mayor, a five-year-old boy at the time he knew Victor's grandparents, begins to tell their story. The account commences in the past tense and yet as the memories recounted start to overtake the speaker he switches into the present. The presence of the past is at its most intense when the two men reach the room in which the grandparents had been hidden. Here, the narration comes to an end as Victor abruptly dismisses the mayor, asking to be left alone for a moment in the room.

Nowhere in the film is the question of witnessing posed in a more highly charged or unsettling way. For at the very moment Victor touches a piece of peeling wallpaper, it in turn touches off a kind of explosion in him (see Figure 3). Or to be more precise, what explodes are disembodied memories, memories belonging to no one, memories no one person seems able to grasp. They are memories, the visual language of the film suggests, that have been walled up and papered over—not only in the room itself but in the Bastien–Gornick family and in French society in general. These memories now explode onto the scene like a traumatic flashback. Suddenly, we are transported back into the past in which another dance is being performed.

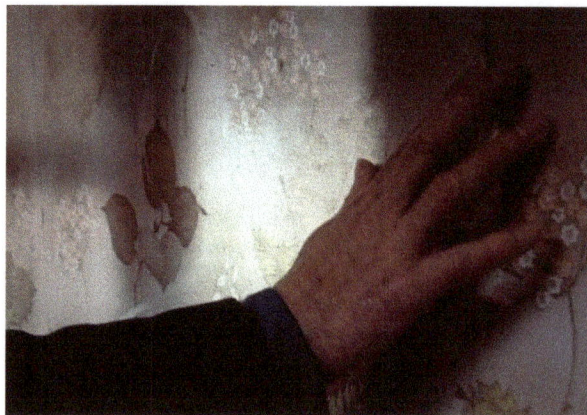

Figure 3. Peeling Wallpaper.

Like the dance of the mother and son at the beginning of the film, this one involving Victor's grandmother and grandfather begins slowly, gently, and lovingly (see Figure 4). The two look deeply into each other's eyes as though for the last time while familiar music plays quietly in the background. Yet, as the music speeds up, the dance partners turn ever more rapidly around each other and the action itself becomes harder and harder for the audience to follow. The film cuts with increasing rapidity between inside and out, between hidden Jews, caged animals, and those who have come to hunt them down. As chaos, terror, and panic spread, a sense of visual disorientation is compounded by ever-increasing levels of acoustic interference. The familiarity of the French language quickly gives way to a confusion of tongues, to linguistic babble that in its turn disintegrates into pure, almost deafening noise. At the center of this wrenchingly violent scene and at the height of its overwhelming chaos, all the audience sees is gravel crushed under foot. All it hears is the grinding of stones, the firing of guns, the growling of dogs, and the incoherent barking of commands (see Figure 5). What began slowly as a couple's turning embrace quickly accelerates into a vertiginous dance of death.

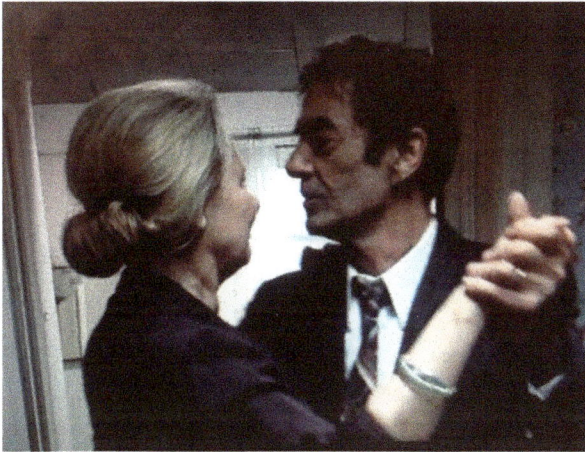

Figure 4. Dance.

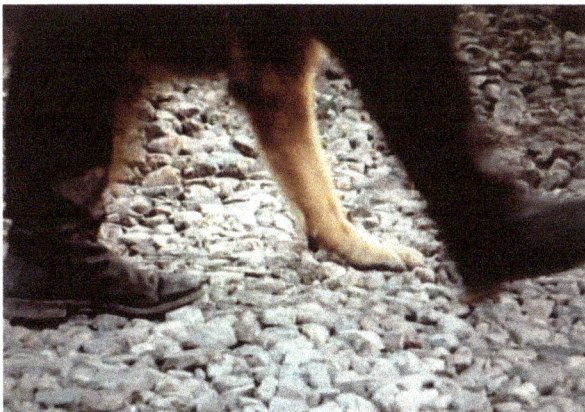

Figure 5. Roundup in Salviac.

This is the dead center of the film, the vortex into which its various perspectives collapse. While the scene eventually shifts away from the stones being crushed underfoot, the sound of their clattering remains in the audience's ears, becoming particularly resonant in a later scene in which memorial stones are the subject of a conversation between Victor's sister and his wife. Christians put flowers on graves, one tells the other, while Jews place stones in memory of their years of wandering in the desert. In the desert, it is said, stones served as path markers, as touchstones, as *points de repère*; they were a way to get one's bearings.

Bearing this scene in mind, let us return to an earlier, closely related one in which the question of Jewish mourning is already posed. In it, Raymonde—or Rivka as she is now called—takes her own grandchildren to a synagogue on Yom Kippur, the day on which, she tells them, Jews remember their dead (see Figure 6). The scene is particularly poignant since we have just learned that Rivka is herself fatally ill. Indeed, at the point she takes her grandchildren to the synagogue for the first and last time, she is positioned at once as one of the mourners and as someone who is herself about to be mourned. Standing in a sense between the living and the dead, Rivka performs a strikingly equivocal act. For at this moment, what she passes on to her grandchildren, or rather to her grandson, is the yellow star marked *juif* which the Jews of occupied France had been made to wear.

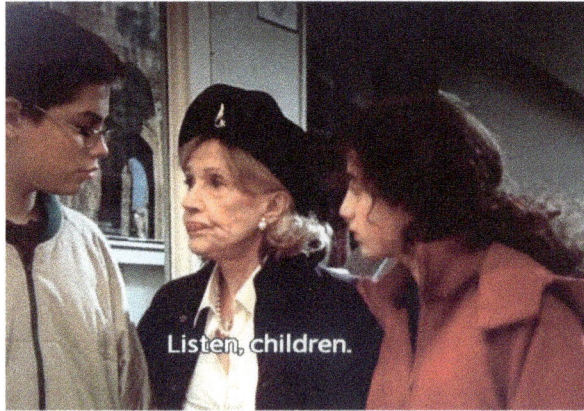

Figure 6. Entrance to Synagogue.

How are we to understand this scene of transmission? What is being passed on? It is the first time Rivka acknowledges to her grandchildren that she is Jewish, doing so in a place symbolizing the survival of Jewish life in France and in view of an Israeli tourist poster hanging conspicuously in the background. Yet, this locus of Jewish survival is a place that seems to have *no other place* in her life—which is perhaps why she only first enters it with the children at a time when she herself is no longer fully among the living, nor quite yet among the dead.

Survival here no longer means simply outliving or living beyond but is associated instead with the liminal space and disjointed time of that which exceeds the very opposition of life and death. It is this threshold of survival on which Rivka will have verged not just at the end but over the last forty years. It is a place unlike any other, a "no place" she will have kept secret not only from others but herself, a place through which family secrets will have secretly been passed. When in the end Rivka gives her grandchildren the Jewish star she had been made to wear, a sign for her of belonging to and with the excluded of French history, she also passes on her own secret, unacknowledged grief.[3]

---

[3] Positioned among the mourners and herself about to be mourned, she is neither simply the subject nor object of grief but more liminally and ambiguously its carrier.

Elsewhere in her life, this grief seems to be stored in evocative objects that fill her apartment (see Figure 7). Yet, strangely enough, no one of them ever appears to stay in her possession for very long, as though the purpose of their incessant exchange were to express the passing of those she could not hold on to, to grieve with each exchange their *ceaseless passing*, to prolong with each new deal her endless grieving.[4] Commenting on his mother's behavior, Clément observes in his memoir, "Toujours acheter, vendre, marchander. Plus pour le geste que le résultat" ['To always be buying, selling, bargaining. More for the gesture than the result'] (Clément 2008, p. 188).

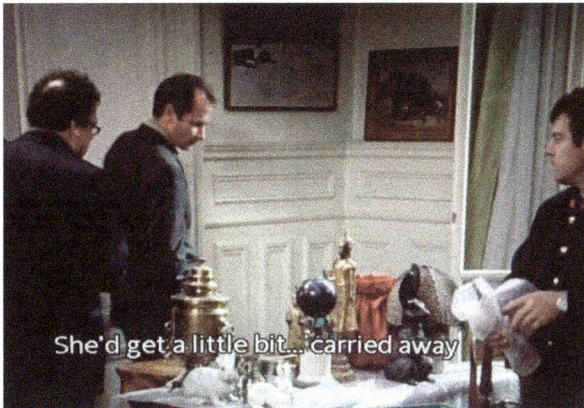

Figure 7. Preparation for Auction.

In the end, we come to see that it is not so much Rivka's secret grief as her secret *way* of grieving that passes in compulsively repeated gestures between generations. Thus, upon her demise, Jean, like his mother, prepares for another auction. Or as Clément reflects in his memoir, "Finalement, en remettant ces objets en vente, je les rends à leurs destination initiale. Ils passent de main en main. C'est bien ainsi, je n'en ai été que le proprietaire momentané" ['Finally in putting these objects up for sale I am returning them to their original destination. They pass from hand to hand. It's good this way. I was never more than the temporary owner'] (Clément 2008, p. 226).

Gitai takes this movement of circulation and exchange one step further. Moving beyond the auctions in which mother and son each in turn take part, he adds a final scene set at the CIVS established in 1999 by the French government in recognition of its responsibility in the deportation and murder of French Jews. During his appointment at the commission, Victor sees a price being placed on everything his maternal grandparents had once owned. Yet, rather than feeling that justice is now finally being served, that the story of his mother's side of the family, kept secret for close to sixty years, is now being publicly aired and officially addressed, Victor seems only to feel increasingly uncomfortable, anxious and overwhelmed (see Figure 8).

---

4   This is in contrast to the Proustian view of memory articulated in the following famous passage from *Swan's Way*: "The past is hidden somewhere outside the realm [of voluntary memory], beyond the reach, of intellect, in some material object . . . which we do not suspect. And as for that object, it depends on chance whether we come upon it or not before we ourselves must die" (Proust 2003, p. 59).

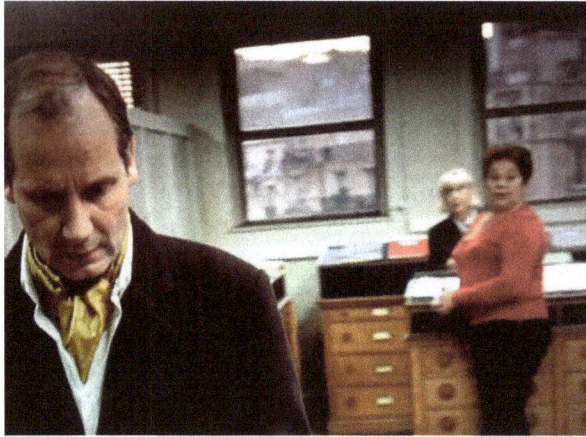

Figure 8. CIVS.

Whereas in the auctions, memory-filled objects were placed in circulation, here it is memories preserved in official documents that are lost almost as quickly and suddenly as they are evoked. Indeed, Victor seems overwhelmed not so much by these fleeting memories themselves *as by their flight in rapid succession*, their abrupt passage conjuring the passing of those he never knew except as the ghosts of his mother's apartment. The disorienting speed at which these memories pass is itself evocative of the earlier scene of the grandparents' arrest. As noted above, this is less a discrete scene than a vertiginously fast-paced, quickly cut montage, less a memory any character in the film is able to access than a sudden explosion of memory fragments. It is this traumatically shattered—and still shattering—scene of her parents' abrupt passing that the mother never witnesses as such but that seems to return in various guises throughout the film and to be rehearsed in the incessant exchange of objects associated with her clandestine way of grieving.

Fleeing from this final encounter with the reparations people and all that it seems inadvertently to touch on, Victor walks down a long hallway, the film's last spoken word *traces* no doubt lingering in his ear. He comes to a halt finally before another open window, where he is left once again to catch his breath, his gaze seemingly fixed on the base of the Eiffel Tower (see Figure 9).

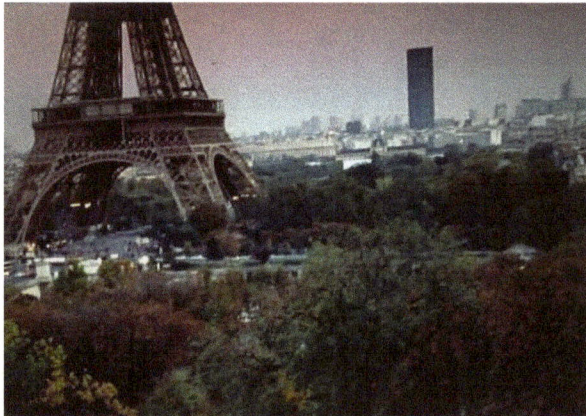

Figure 9. View of Eiffel Tower from CIVS.

Why do his eyes not follow the ascent of the tower's famously tapering lines? Why does the filmmaker, a trained architect, prevent him as well as the viewer from looking upward, from experiencing the expansive sense of relief associated with such a skyward gaze? Particularly in view of the television and radio transmissions of the Barbie trial which play such a central role in the opening moments of the film, it is important to recall how the initial lines of the tower were extended and further elongated by the addition of a broadcast antenna in 1957. Not only is this antenna pointedly kept out of view in the shot in question but as the eye is made to dwell exclusively on the tower's base, the viewer is reminded of the pent-up energies accumulating below. Such energies, it is suggested, are denied more traditional modes of transmission, modes associated with the radio and television signals broadcast over public airwaves from the antenna above. Yet, what remains below, remaining like grief denied successful translation into juridical grievance or financial compensation, is not simply lost in transmission. Remaining unconsciously insistent, it passes instead via other, more subliminal channels.

After a long pause, the camera eventually turns from this view. Yet, as though to suggest that something grievous will have happened in the meantime, it is no longer the protagonist's perspective the audience shares. Victor has himself somehow vanished from the scene and it is now the withdrawing camera that returns alone, moving visibly backwards down a long corridor (see Figure 10).

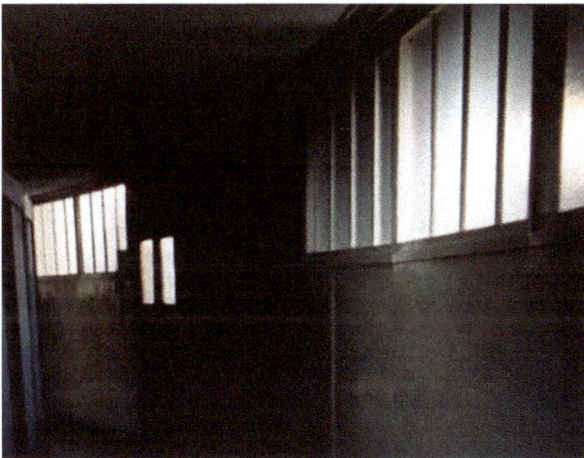

Figure 10. CIVS Corridor.

Retreating from the daylight that had entered through the open window where Victor is last seen, and withdrawing from all the other sources of inner illumination, the camera's eye closes in the end, fading like the scene itself into total darkness. The ending seems to equate these last glimmers of light with the invisible yet hauntingly palpable traces of another family legacy, a secret grief secretly passed from mother to son and beyond.

This grieving, unwittingly disowned from generation to generation, is comparable to the objects Jean puts back in circulation, returning them, as Clément says, to their *destination initiale*. This grief, without object and without end, is in dialogue with the Barbie trial against which the film is set and with which it begins. The "abyss of mourning", still open within the family, bears witness to the failure of the trial itself to translate grief into grievance.

Reading the family story back onto the trial, we come to see the endless grieving it performs as an unaddressed grievance, as a symptom of the many failures of the trial: among them, its confusion of the Resistance and the Jewish victims; its dilution of the category of crimes against humanity;[5] and its rather outrageous implication that a democratic state cannot commit such crimes[6]. The "no place" of Rivka's grief may thus be said to bear witness to a certain *non-lieu* of the trial—the term *non-lieu* referring in this case less to a dismissal of charges than to the confusing way in which they were brought. This confusion ended up pitting the various plaintiffs against each other and gave the defense attorney Jacques Vergès the opportunity to present what Alice Kaplan has aptly referred to as a Pandora's box version of crimes against humanity, a version where one crime would effectively call up all the others, making them equally intolerable and putting them into competition with each other so that justice always seems hypocritical[7].

Kaplan summarizes this state of confusion in her excellent introduction to the English translation of Alain Finkielkraut's *Remembering in Vain: The Klaus Barbie Trial and Crimes Against Humanity* published in 1992:

> The Barbie trial was, for France, like an abreaction in psychoanalysis, a single relived piece of trauma that brings the other buried pieces back to life. When abreaction works, it produces a catharsis and cure. Finkielkraut would contend that the Barbie trial was the very opposite: that lots of time and work went into avoiding what should have been central; that with avoidance and denial came the release of accumulated social toxins. (Finkielkraut 1992, p. xvii)

Kaplan's potent metaphor returns us in the end to Felman's description of the law as a necessarily flawed containment strategy. "The law," she says, "tries to contain the trauma and to translate it into legal-conscious terminology, thus reducing its strange interruption. Uncannily, however, while the law strives to contain the trauma, it often is in fact the trauma that takes over and whose surreptitious logic in the end reclaims the trial" (Felman 2002, p. 5). If there is a difference between Kaplan's and Felman's perspectives, it perhaps lies in the latter's sense that failure is not incidental to the law, is not avoidable in its engagement with historical trauma. Such failures for Felman instead mark its very fault lines, its constitutive openness to the supplement of what she calls *literary justice*. One of the most provocative questions she asks in *The Juridical Unconscious* is whether literature (and film) in their supplementary relationship to the law might do justice to the trauma in a way the law does not, or cannot.

In her most sweeping response to this question, Felman writes: "Literature is a dimension of concrete embodiment and a language of infinitude that, in contrast to the language of the law, encapsulates not closure but precisely what in a given legal case refuses to be closed and cannot be closed. It is to this refusal of the trauma to be closed that literature does justice" (Felman 2002, p. 8).

Where does this leave us then with regard to *One Day You'll Understand?* I would argue that Clément, in re-opening the crypt of his initial memoir, transforms the work of mourning he had sought to accomplish there into something much larger. Turning it, with his writing partner, Serge Moati, into a screenplay and then with Amos Gitai into a film, Clément repositions it in the very margin of legal closure, on the brink of the abyss that underlies the law. Such repositioning turns the memoir itself into an interminable work of mourning, a work that in many essential respects escapes him and in the most concrete ways no longer belongs to him. It is no doubt for this reason that he opens the sequel to the memoir with the words of another. His sister, the philosopher Catherine Clément,

---

[5] The court's decision meant that deportations of the Jews and of the members of the Resistance were legally equivalent acts (Douglas 2001, p. 195).

[6] Whereas at Nuremberg crimes against humanity were essentially enfolded into war crimes, the Barbie trial, "in a stunning inversion, did just the opposite: war crimes were enfolded into crimes against humanity, which now, in the interpretation of French courts, became a master category embracing a wide variety of wartime transgressions". (Douglas 2001, p. 195).

[7] The endless grieving enacted in the film would thus have as its juridical equivalent the re-opening of one wound through another, the simultaneous "calling up," as Kaplan puts it, of all the others through the one crime (Finkielkraut 1992, p. xxvi).

Humanities **2017**, *6*, 93

tells him, "Tu crois en avoir fini ... tu te trompes, on n'en a jamais fini" ['You think you're finished with it. You're wrong. One is never finished with it'] (Clément 2008, p. 273).

Conflicts of Interest: The author declares no conflict of interest.

References

Clément, Jerôme. 2008. *Plus Tard, tu Comprendras Suivi de Maintenant, Je Sais.* Paris: Editions Grasset & Fasquelle.

Douglas, Lawrence. 2001. *The Memory of Judgment: Making Law and History in the Trials of the Holocaust.* New Haven: Yale University Press.

Felman, Shoshana. 2002. *The Juridical Unconscious: Trials and Traumas in the Twentieth Century.* Cambridge: Harvard University Press.

Finkielkraut, Alain. 1992. *Remembering in Vain: The Klaus Barbie Trial and Crimes against Humanity.* New York: Columbia University Press.

Gitai, Amos. 2008. *One Day You'll Understand [Plus Tard, tu Comprendras].* Paris: Agav Films.

Proust, Marcel. 2003. *In Search of Lost Time, Volume 1: Swann's Way.* New York: Modern Library.

Rottenberg, Elizabeth. 2004. The Juridical Unconscious: Trials and Traumas in the Twentieth Century (review). *MLN* 119: 1098–103. [CrossRef]

Rousso, Henry. 1991. *The Vichy Syndrome: History and Memory in France since 1944.* Cambridge: Harvard University Press.

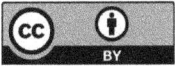

humanities

MDPI

Article

In Transit: Sebald, Trauma, and Cinema

Allen Meek

School of English and Media Studies, Massey University, Palmerston North 4442, New Zealand;
A.Meek@massey.ac.nz

Received: 13 October 2017; Accepted: 14 December 2017; Published: 18 December 2017

Abstract: Because Sebald's books are preoccupied with historical catastrophe, particularly the Holocaust, critical commentaries have often interpreted them in terms of the transmission of traumatic memory. But this stress on the temporal relay from past to present and future generations has drawn attention away from the emphasis on space and travel in Sebald's work. In order to address this gap in Sebald criticism, this essay discusses three films that adapt and respond to Sebald's work: *Patience (After Sebald)* (directed by Grant Gee, 2012), *Terezin* (directed by Daniel Blaufuks, 2010) and *Austerlitz* (directed by Stan Neumann, 2015). Because of the cinema's constant movement between images and places, these films allow us to see more clearly the aspects of Sebald's writings concerned with traveling and making connections between different archival spaces. The journeys in Sebald's books and in these films inspired by them go beyond human life worlds to include non-human creatures, and beyond the realms of the living to include those inhabited by the dead. This suspension of the boundary between life and death, along with the restless movement from place to place, creates a relationship to memory and history that cannot be limited to the model of traumatic transmission.

Keywords: Sebald; trauma; postmemory; cinema; Holocaust

It does not seem to me, Austerlitz added, that we understand the laws governing the return of the past, but I feel more and more as if time did not exist at all, only various spaces interlocking according to the rules of a higher form of stereometry, between which the living and the dead can move back and forth as they like, and the longer I think about it the more it seems to me that we who are still alive are unreal in the eyes of the dead, that only occasionally, in certain lights and atmospheric conditions, do we appear in their field of vision (Sebald 2001, p. 185).

The passage cited above, from W.G. Sebald's *Austerlitz*, is spoken in the closing moments of Stan Neumann's film of the novel, suggesting that the director presents it as in some sense a conclusion not only of, but also about, the film. Could the various interlocking spaces referred to in this passage describe the different images and sequences that compose a cinematic montage? Does the cinema allow the living and the dead to move freely between different spaces? The cinema, wrote Walter Benjamin, opens up "a vast and unsuspected field of action" (Benjamin 2002, p. 117): it allows the juxtaposition of multiple spaces and the possibility of unlimited movement through those spaces. If we read this passage from *Austerlitz* as a description of cinema, then that movement extends from the worlds of the living to those of the dead. Benjamin goes on: "With the close-up, space expands; with slow motion, movement is extended" (Benjamin 2002, p. 117). Does film not also transport us to places where the dead, as well as the living, continue to make gestures and move about? This paradox is given a dramatic expression in Sebald's novel, in which the character Jacques Austerlitz has a slow-motion version made of a documentary so that he can search for an image of his mother, who died in Auschwitz.

The following discussion reconsiders some of Sebald's narratives and use of images in light of three films that adapt and respond to his work: *Patience (After Sebald)* (directed by Grant Gee (Gee 2012)), *Terezin* (directed by Daniel Blaufuks (Blaufuks 2010b) and *Austerlitz* (directed by Stan Neumann (Neumann 2015)). These cinematic versions of Sebald allow us to see more clearly the ways that his narratives are continually moving through different spaces inhabited by the living and the dead.

Influential writings on literature and cinema by Shoshana Felman, Cathy Caruth and Marianne Hirsch have focused on the transmission of traumatic memory through testimony. According to these theorists the overwhelming impact of violent and catastrophic events is registered in memory in the form of indelible traces that can be transmitted to others as an authentic experience of history. In this way trauma, although it may not be accessible to an individual's conscious understanding, can be recovered and become part of the collective memory of a particular group. In the writings of these critics historical trauma serves as the basis of identification with the sufferer, thereby bearing witness to a previously unacknowledged truth about the past. Traumatic experiences can be the cause of pathological conditions and behaviors and trauma theory invites us to enter "inside" this traumatized worldview. It is hardly surprising, then, that Sebald's work has invited critical commentary using trauma as an interpretive frame. Sebald's narratives about historical catastrophe feature characters that are disoriented and despairing as a result of surviving emigration, exile, war and genocide. These characters bear witness to a traumatic experience of history, their voices recorded in documentary style, accompanied by photographs of people, events, places and artifacts that appear to lend further authenticity to their testimony. The reader is invited to identify with these characters and experience their reality, with its melancholy heaviness, feelings of loss and sense of being lost.

The emphasis placed by these critics on identification, transmission, authenticity and truth, however, is less useful for understanding the intricate weaving of intertextual references and layering of genres in Sebald's books. Sebald's mixing of travelogue, history, testimony and archival materials suggests the genre of documentary, yet his texts also combine fact with fiction, authentic evidence with fake documents, narrative progression with obscure meditations and digressions. To interpret the elaborate construction of these texts as symptomatic of a pathological anxiety or obsession would be to willfully ignore their deliberate irony and ambiguity. This dimension of crafting is precisely what makes these texts "literary." The following discussion proposes that they are also usefully understood as "cinematic": Sebald's books recall the cinema in their restless movement between distant times and places, their juxtaposition of multiple spaces, and their suggestions of unexpected connections between disparate events and environments.

Rather than allowing us to experience historical trauma from the "inside," Sebald's multidirectional journeys and histories suggest a more permeable and porous boundary between past and present, life and death. The intrusive force of trauma cannot account for the diverse ways that memory is actively explored, carefully re-presented and intensively mediated in Sebald's work. His montage of image and text is not only full of parallel narratives and verbal echoes but includes forms of visual patterning that have influenced contemporary artists and filmmakers. There is a graphic dimension to Sebald's books that, along with the attention to architectural spaces and natural landscapes, makes the visual as important as the verbal. This mosaic construction does not easily lend itself to the notion of transmission of, or identification with, traumatic memory: instead it appears to continually defer and displace such identifications through spatial movement and visual correspondences.

Too often commentaries on Sebald explain his texts as embodying and communicating trauma at the expense of considering their complex spatial organization. For example, in her commentary on the passage from *Austerlitz* cited at the beginning of this essay, Luisa Banki writes: "What this image entails is the threatening dissolution of order into chaos . . . identical with the danger of being overwhelmed by (actualised) traumatic memories" (Banki 2012, p. 43). Banki's commentary is consistent with psychoanalytic and psychotherapeutic accounts of trauma in which the individual subject is overwhelmed by specific memories of events so painful or incomprehensible at the time of their occurrence that they were not registered by the conscious mind. The memories of the events then return to the subject in later life in the form of nightmares, flashbacks, and pathological symptoms and behaviors. However, if we reconsider the particular passage that Banki cites from the novel, we see that the image is not one of chaos and dissolution but of "various spaces interlocking according to . . . rules" (Sebald 2001, p. 185). What the character Jacques Austerlitz imagines is that these laws or rules that govern our relation to the past have to do with a spatial organization beyond our comprehension. Austerlitz "feels" this spatiality is not bound by the logic of linear temporality or to the distinction between life and death. Although this image of a "higher form of stereometry" (Sebald 2001, p. 185) is voiced by a character who can be understood as traumatized, this passage from the novel also suggests a self-reflexive commentary on the mixture of travelogue, history, testimony, and archival images in Sebald's fictions.

Continuing to read Sebald according to the logic of traumatic memory may be distracting us from better understanding the spatial organization of his narratives in which past and present, living and dead, co-exist in a non-temporal relationship. Trauma theory stresses the sudden and unexpected intrusion of the past into the present and the historical transmission of collective memory. In the Preface to her edited collection *Trauma: Explorations in Memory*, Caruth writes of the problem of "how to understand the nature of the suffering, without eliminating the force and truth of the reality that trauma survivors face and quite often try to transmit to us" (Caruth 1995a, p. vii). This emphasis on the particular truth of traumatic memory, along with its transmission from survivor to witness, links it to the collective identification with an authentic experience of history. In her Introduction, Caruth goes on to explain that this experience has a specific structure: "the event is not assimilated or experienced fully at the time, but only belatedly, in its repeated *possession* of the one who experiences it" (Caruth 1995b, p. 4). Caruth's theory of traumatic memory may at first appear to precisely describe the narrative about Jacques Austerlitz, who rediscovers his origins as a European Jew by recovering a memory of his arrival at Liverpool station as part of the *Kindertransport* that bought Jewish refugee children to England in World War II: his obsession with train stations can be explained in terms of this experience that he was not able to fully comprehend at the time of its occurrence. Yet Sebald's journeys do not only move between past and present but also make connections between multiple and diverse locations. In this way they divert us away from identification with a single historical truth or the experience of a particular group.

The proliferation of different spaces in Sebald's works and the often unexpected routes, passageways, and detours that connect them is foregrounded in the films about his works. This is particularly true of *Patience (After Sebald)*, the subtitle of which is "A Walk through *Rings of Saturn*": the film re-enacts the walk through East Anglia described in Sebald's book but also "walks" the viewer through the book itself, using the guidance of experts on Sebald's work and associates of the author. The film uses digital mapping to show the dense complexity of connections between different places mentioned in the book. Movement between multiple locations also characterizes Neumann's film of *Austerlitz*, in which the director revisits the different places described in the novel and also talks about his own fascination with, and autobiographical connections to, the narrative. The idea of architecture and nature as archival spaces characterizes both *Patience* and the film version of *Austerlitz*. By repeating the journeys in Sebald's books, these films inquire into the ways that memory is embedded in human and natural environments. Sebald's writings themselves often use the strategy of following in the footsteps of others; for example, in his first book *Vertigo* he repeats a journey to Riva made earlier by Franz Kafka (Sebald 1999, pp. 141–67). Just as Sebald follows the trajectories of other writers, filmmakers have attempted to reproduce the journeys described in Sebald's books. Using the interpretive frames suggested by trauma theory, we might see these repetitions as symptomatic of a transmission of traumatic memory, even as a compulsive response to the historical traumas invoked in the novels. Howevert although walking and traveling can certainly be seen as compulsive activities, they also suggest active exploration, making choices based on impulse and curiosity, and a deliberate agency in terms of pursuing memory. Sebald's journeys not only allow encounters with the traumatic past, they also lead us to discover new configurations of memory and history and new constellations of disparate worlds.

1. Sebald and *Shoah*

Restless traveling can be seen as a means of avoiding painful memories. Journeys can also deliberately return to places where calamities have occurred. Learning to recognize the legacies of the past in landscapes, cityscapes, and imagescapes demands a complex model of space and place that goes beyond the specific temporal structure of traumatic memory. Because Sebald's journeys are so persistently preoccupied with the legacies of historical catastrophe, and particularly of the Jewish Holocaust, Mark M. Anderson compares his works to Claude Lanzmann's famous documentary film *Shoah*, in which Lanzmann revisits the sites of the deportations and mass murder and interviews survivors and witnesses in the places where these atrocities occurred (Anderson 2003, pp. 106–7). In Lanzmann's film, as in Sebald's writings, cities, towns and landscapes suggest forms of memory and forgetting that exist alongside the individual testimony of the survivor witness.

As with Sebald's work, interpretations of Lanzmann's film have been dominated by the idea of traumatic transmission. This interpretive frame, however, has tended to neglect the various ways that the film traverses and dwells in different places. For example, Shoshana Felman writes that "*Shoah* is a film made exclusively of testimonies" (Felman and Laub 1992, p. 205). However, it is also a film about places and journeys; thus she comments: "Traveling between the living and the dead and moving to and fro between the different places and different voices in the film, the filmmaker is continuously—though discretely—present" (Felman and Laub 1992, p. 216). This sounds remarkably similar to Jacques Austerlitz's description of the spaces between which the living and the dead can move back and forth as they like, until Felman explains this movement more specifically in terms of an "inside" and "outside". Lanzmann, writes Felman, "takes us an a journey whose aim precisely is to cross the boundary, first from the outside world to the inside of the Holocaust, and back from the inside of the Holocaust to the outside world" (Felman and Laub 1992, p. 238). For Felman the point of Lanzmann's journey is to enter into the traumatic experience of the victim/survivor and to transmit this to the witness. The inside/outside polarity imposed on Lanzmann's journey to the sites of the Nazi genocide reinforces the identification with the victim that drives his film. In Sebald's writings, however, this identification is more indirect and more complexly mediated. His fictions and the films they have inspired suggest ways to think about memory, testimony, and archival images that transcend the model of traumatic transmission. In Sebald the boundaries between the insider's and outsider's experience are less important than the interconnections between different life worlds and scenes of death and decay.

The ways that movements through spaces and journeys to and from places are imagined is shaped by identifications with the groups that inhabit these spaces and places. Sebald, the non-Jewish German, creates the character Jacques Austerlitz who grows up in Wales unaware of his Jewish origins in Czechoslovakia. Whereas Sebald left his native Germany and pursued a career as an émigré academic in England, the assimilated French Jew Lanzmann went to Germany in 1947 to lecture on German philosophy at Berlin University. Lanzmann subsequently travelled to East Germany and to Israel, where he rediscovered his Jewish identity. For Felman, Lanzmann's journey in *Shoah* is about the struggle to bear witness from inside the Holocaust and through an identification with the Jewish victims and survivors (many of whom he finds in Israel). The witness, writes Felman, "embodies the return of the dead" (Felman and Laub 1992, p. 257). Trauma is always linked to the idea of recovery of what was lost or missing, and is then aligned with identification with a specific group. In Austerlitz's image of the living and the dead moving freely through various spaces, however, nothing is necessarily lost or recovered or transmitted. Instead there is a sense that the living and the dead co-exist, even if they do not always recognize each other. The living and the dead in Sebald's books never cohere into a single community. Rather they appear to encounter each other or pass each other by, like the inhabitants of some vast necropolis.

This sense of the co-existence of the living and the dead is memorably conveyed in *Austerlitz* in the title character's attempts to recover an image of his lost mother by repeatedly watching a slow-motion version of the Nazi documentary about Theresienstadt camp. Austerlitz can never be sure if he has found an image of his mother, as he has no conscious memory of her and has only a few old photographs upon which to base his idea of her appearance. This film, which shows a world inhabited by the dead, is also a false image of life in the camp fabricated by the Nazis and therefore cannot stand as an authentic record of past events. What it does incontestably show is a specific place, Theresienstadt, whose inhabitants have all been murdered.

2. Sebald and Cinema

Sebald's books, with their intensive use of photographs and other images and their descriptions of journeys and places, seem to invite the designation "cinematic." At various moments in Sebald's novels specific films are mentioned or discussed.[1] In an essay on cinema in Sebald's work Mattias Frey compares Sebald's model of composition to cinematic montage, specifically as it is developed in the films of Alexander Kluge, Jean-Luc Godard and Alain Resnais (Frey 2007, pp. 231–2). Frey also develops a detailed analysis of a sequence of photographs in Austerlitz that record moving through the Theresienstadt camp (Frey 2007, pp. 233–36). This exploration of the camp as it stands today appears as an actual film sequence in Neumann's film of *Austerlitz*.

Austerlitz the novel includes visits to two now uninhabited Nazi camps: Breendonk in Belgium and Theresienstadt in Czechoslovakia. The image of returning to the ruins of the camps is used in both Resnais' *Night and Fog* and Lanzmann's *Shoah*. In Resnais' film the camera tracks across the deserted space of the camps, alternating with various archival photographs and documentary films from the period of the genocide. Lanzmann avoids archival images, but juxtaposes sequences shot in the now empty camps with the testimony of survivors and witnesses. Sebald's own montage of photographs taken at Theresienstadt doubtless makes a deliberate and self-conscious reference to these two iconic Holocaust documentaries. Film scholar Joshua Hirsch describes the opening sequence of *Night and Fog*, showing the barbed wire fences of Auschwitz, as situated at the border "between the present and the past, between the outside world and the inner world of the concentration camp" (Hirsch 2004, p. 48). Like Felman's reading of *Shoah*, he reads Resnais' film as transmitting traumatic memory. However, in Sebald's fictions any image, object, or place potentially becomes a threshold across which the narrator moves into another archival space. There is no inside or outside determined specifically by the experience or memory of the Holocaust.

Sebald's various references to films in his books, including those by Resnais and Kluge, and his use of photographs to document his journeys suggests that he at least partly intended an analogy between writer and filmmaker. This analogy both reinforces and exceeds the "traumatic" interpretation of Sebald's work. Photographs and film images preserve actual traces of people, things, places and events that are no longer present. In this way they suggest a strong analogy with the conception of traumatic memory as a literal trace of the past preserved outside conscious memory (Meek 2010, pp. 35–8). Indeed Amit Pinchevski has proposed that the audio-visual archive "might be considered the technological unconscious . . . of what came to be known as 'trauma theory'" (Pinchevski 2011, p. 258), giving the example of the Fortunoff Video Archive for Holocaust Testimonies at Yale University, which became the basis for subsequent commentary and analysis by scholars such as Geoffrey Hartman, Dori Laub, and Lawrence Langer. Pinchevski argues that the location of specific moments when traumatic memories intrude into the survivor's testimony could only be analyzed because of "the ability to pause, rewind, and replay" (Pinchevski 2011, p. 259) videotape. The very notion that testimony could transmit a traumatic memory from survivor to witness was premised on the technological capabilities of recording, archiving, and replaying movement and sound.

---

[1]　See for example *Vertigo* (Sebald 1999, pp. 150–52), which describes Kafka's visit to the cinema; *The Emigrants* (Sebald 1996, p. 17), where a home move is compared to a sequence from Werner Herzog's *Kaspar Hauser*; *The Rings of Saturn* (Sebald 1998, p. 103), which describes a BBC documentary about Roger Casement; and *Austerlitz*, which includes references to Leni Riefenstahl's *Triumph of the Will* (p. 169) and Alain Resnais' documentary about the Bibliotheque Nationale, *Tout le Mémoire du Monde* (p. 261).

Felman's and Hirsch's comparison of the journeys undertaken by Lanzmann and Resnais as moving from the outside to the inside of the Holocaust could also describe the process of recording, replaying and editing by which the filmmaker collects and shapes the materials. In this sense Sebald's character Austerlitz, an amateur photographer (like Sebald himself), becomes a filmmaker as he repeatedly watches and pauses the slow-motion version of the Nazi documentary of Thereienstadt. But if *Shoah* and the Fortunoff Video Archive allowed researchers to replay moments of testimony on order to recover moments of traumatic transmission, Sebald's approach to the audiovisual archive is quite different: when Austerlitz replays the slow-motion version of the Thereienstadt film, it is unclear whether anything is recovered or transmitted.

The notion of the transmission of trauma derives from psychological studies of second-generation experiences of the Holocaust: the trauma suffered by the parents was in some ways transmitted to the children, not by what was directly said but by what remained unsaid or was expressed in pathological behaviors (Hirsch 2004, p. 17). This transmission across generations is also relevant to larger claims about post-Holocaust Jewish identity. Again, however, Sebald's fictions do not easily conform to this account of traumatic transmission: first, the storyteller is a fabrication of the author and his statements are often composed of words borrowed from other texts; second, the process of identification is more indirect and complex because the Jewish character has no direct experience of the historical events of the Holocaust and his testimony is further mediated by the non-Jewish narrator. In Sebald's writings and their cinematic adaptations the movement between the worlds of the dead and the living does not always follow the logic of a collective identification. Rather, the present world of landscapes, buildings, artifacts, and images forms a potentially infinite series of archival spaces. The journey does not arrive at a final destination or a sense of belonging to a specific community of victims, survivors, or witnesses. The tension between archival images and living testimony that informs Lanzmann's intentions in *Shoah* does not apply to Sebald's works. All archival spaces, whether real places or documentary records, become sites of a possible encounter with an elusive past.

2.1. Patience (After Sebald)

A sense of an almost global meditation on historical catastrophe is conveyed in Grant Gee's film *Patience (After Sebald)*, subtitled "A Walk through *Rings of Saturn*." The film is largely composed of interviews with a variety of interpreters and associates of Sebald and with artists who have been inspired by his work. The film superimposes these interviews and commentaries on images and passages of text from *The Rings of Saturn*, images of the places described in the journey around East Anglia described in the novel, and archival images and footage related to the various events and histories described in Sebald's text, including World War II bombing raids, silk worm farming, and fishing at Lowestoft. The film, then, carries the dense intertextuality of the book into an overtly hyper-textual film, where archival images and footage, verbal text, interviews, and films of actual places are continually juxtaposed and superimposed. To reinforce the sense that the film is a journey, there are shots from the point of view of the walker looking down on his legs and feet moving through the landscape, arms shown rowing a boat across glistening water, and atmospheric shots of places on the journey. The effect is that as we experience moving through the landscape we are also progressing through the text and images in the book. Marina Warner comments in the film that just as Sebald's "walks meander, his mind meanders and the pattern of the structure of the book meanders" (Gee 2012).

There is also an irony in this strategy, as interviewee Robert Macfarlane explains about his own attempt to reproduce the actual journey that forms the basis of the narrative in *The Rings of Saturn*: "It soon became obvious to me that the way to write about Sebald (I was wrong in this assumption) was to follow him, was to footstep in his foot-stepping of earlier feet and turn his own method back upon himself" (Gee 2012). Unfortunately this mimetic strategy produces unpredictable results: "I re-walked most of *The Rings of Saturn* walk and I really wanted it to be a grey day and it wasn't a grey day it was a bright day" (Gee 2012). Instead of immersing himself in Sebaldian melancholy, Macfarlane finds himself enjoying a refreshing swim in the sea. Should we take this anecdote as an ironic commentary on the folly of trying to recreate Sebald's book in Gee's film? The multitude of voices that offer commentary in *Patience* does contrast with the slow, meditative—almost hypnotic—effect of Sebald's prose. One senses Gee as a filmmaker trying to compensate for this somewhat chatty quality of the film with his use of faded black and white images, ambient piano music, and the deep voice (not Sebald's own but no doubt chosen to resemble his) that reads passages from the book.

Patience is composed of zooms on digital maps, grainy close-ups of printed texts, shots from moving trains and car windows tracking through landscapes and towns, the leisurely pace of the cutting mimicking the slow, meditative quality of Sebald's texts. The drama of historical events is never shown but felt as an absence, embodied in objects and places. In terms of cinema history, *Patience* returns to the style of the first Lumiere shorts, their still frames and long takes animated only by grass or leaves of trees moving gently in the wind, or the surface of waters shimmering with light. Sometimes a bird crosses the sky, a pedestrian crosses a street, or a car drives past the unmoving camera. In other places archival footage is modified through slow-motion effects, or there are slow zooms on still images. Images constantly merge into each other through dissolves and superimpositions. This slowness is only occasionally disrupted by a montage of rapid cuts used to convey psychological disorientation and distress. Just as Sebald's texts often resemble a report illustrated by dull black-and-white photographs, *Patience* uses all of the standard tropes of documentary—interviews, location shots, archival footage—and emphasizes their low-key production system and melancholy ambience. By attempting to reproduce the visual style of Sebald's texts, *Patience* reveals Sebald's profound debt to cinema as a visual language.

From the beginning of the film there is an emphasis on digital mapping in the work of artists such as Barbara Hui, who have tried to show the multiple links between the actual places included in Sebald's journey and all of the other places that are mentioned in the text. Indeed *The Rings of Saturn* superimposes a global history of catastrophe on the relatively small territory covered in Sebald's actual walk around East Anglia. Occasionally the film makes use of what looks like Google Earth. Sebald openly discusses his own resistance to computers and the idiocy of those who only research sitting in front of their screens. He stresses the necessity of taking actual journeys to real places in order to encounter true remnants, traces, and documents from the past. In its worst moments the film has a tendency to overload Sebald's solitary, reticent journeys with verbal commentary and technical effects, turning his meditations on time and place into something more akin to contemporary Internet-assisted tourism.

One of the more compelling insights in the film derives from Lise Patt's comparison of an image from the book showing piles of dead fish with another that appears a few pages later portraying victims of the Nazi death camps. This element of visual patterning leads her to comment: "He's become very, very important for contemporary artists, I think. And for that reason we have to reconsider and think of him as both a writer and an artist" (Gee 2012). This sense that Sebald may be an influential artist as well as writer resonates with the filmmaker's mission to turn Sebald's novel into an audiovisual text. For *Patience* is not just a documentary about Sebald's book, but a film that mimics, engages with, and extends both the narrative and visual dimensions of Sebald's work. *Patience*, then, brings out the visual-spatial dimensions of Sebald's text in ways that complicate the emphasis in Sebald commentary on trauma. For example, beyond the visual homology, how should we understand the comparison between dead fish in Lowestoft and dead humans at Belsen? There is certainly no moral equivalence being suggested between these two events, and yet Sebald does continually move back and forth between human catastrophe and the suffering of non-human creatures.

The connection between disparate events through pattern formation is further illuminated later in the film by artist Barbara Hui, who explains:

> Sir Thomas Browne is a very important figure for Sebald in this book. Thomas Browne was a seventeenth century physician/theologian/philosopher/poet and talks about this Quincunx which is this pattern which consists of five nodes essentially and five lines between them, and the notion being that this pattern exists everywhere in nature, sort of

like a primitive network. And it's sort of a very khabbalistic, premodern notion of seeing pattern in the world. And Sebald I think also in his writing is looking for these sorts of patterns, how they occur in historical events and connections between people. (Gee 2012)

Could Browne's Quincunx pattern be another name for the "higher form of stereometry" (Sebald 2001, p. 185) mentioned by Jacques Austerlitz? The patterning that allows us to make visual connections between the diverse images in Sebald's texts serves as a graphic language that traverses the usual boundaries between human and animal, past and present, life and death. This pattern formation thus recalls archaic ways of thinking, or mystical traditions such as the Kabbalah, while also corresponding to modern audiovisual languages such as cinematic montage and digital manipulations of the image.

Perhaps the most profound moment in the film comes in Adam Phillips's discussion of the melancholy temperament:

> In this tradition of melancholy it's as though these people, people who feel this, are people who feel some inexplicable sense of loss. And they're people who try and locate this in history—as in, why am I feeling so fundamentally at a loss and so unattached? And it's as though the history gives you some sort of story about this but the feeling is somehow that there's been some catastrophe that can't be located and that one is living in the aftermath of that catastrophe. (Gee 2012)

This understanding of melancholy usefully relates Sebald's work to the notion of historical trauma at the same time as it differentiates it from Caruth's trauma theory or Marianne Hirsch's notion of postmemory, which tend to be exclusively preoccupied with specific events such as the bombing of Hiroshima or the Holocaust. Although the Holocaust features prominently in Sebald's writings, it is seldom isolated from other historical catastrophes. Marina Warner comments in the film on "his main preoccupation with how the genocidal wars of the twentieth century were foreshadowed by the Victorian Imperial wars" (Gee 2012). This statement is particularly true of *The Rings of Saturn*, which includes a long section on the Belgian genocide in the Congo, but these events resonate in sections of *Austerlitz* also. The narrator's first encounter with Austerlitz in the train station at Antwerp leads to an extended meditation on the bizarre architecture constructed in Belgium during the period of its colonial rule in Africa.

2.2. Terezin

The interconnections in Sebald's writings between various historical catastrophes are also prompted by the deliberate ambiguity that surrounds the images that appear in his texts. In a conversation with Christian Scholz, Sebald muses on his proclivity for finding images "enclosed in old books that one buys ... in antique shops or thrift shops." He comments further: "I've always noticed that an enormous appeal emanates from these images; a demand on the viewer to tell stories or to imagine what one could tell, by starting with these pictures" (Scholz 2007, p. 104). He goes on to link this attraction to archaic conceptions of life and death:

> I believe that the black-and-white photograph, or rather the gray zones in the black-and-white photograph, stand for this territory that is located between death and life. In the archaic imagination it was usually the case that there was not only life and then death, as we assume today, but rather that in between there was this vast no-man's-land where people were permanently wandering around and where one did not know exactly how long one had to stay there ... (Scholz 2007, p. 108)

Sebald's novels re-present numerous photographs and other visual documents, including forgeries and fakes. It is the disjunction between the ambiguity that surrounds the image and the desire of the viewer to emotionally connect with it or to discover in it some previously undisclosed truth that creates the drifting, elusive effect of Sebald's narratives. Readers bring to his texts their own histories and memories and the desire to find in them a meaningful link with the past.

One such reader is Daniel Blaufuks, who made a short film inspired by images that are described in *Austerlitz*. Blaufuks is an artist who explores audiovisual media technologies and archives and their relation to personal and cultural memory. His works often address issues of travel, displacement, and statelessness and his research methods resonate strongly with Sebald's work. Blaufuks's Jewish German grandparents fled Nazi Germany to settle in Lisbon in 1936. In an interview he comments: "I like the idea of transmission, and that you give a different meaning to an unrelated snapshot someone did, perhaps with no further intentions. To change the status of the image that you find in the garbage, or flea market or, for that matter, in an archive" (Blaufuks 2012, p. 31).

Transmission, as a conveying of memory across space and time, also makes it possible to transform the significance of documents and to bestow new meanings on images. Although Blaufuks directly identifies himself with the victims of the Holocaust through his own family history, he also enlarges the idea of traumatic transmission to include Sebaldian aleatory effects. In his book *Terezin* Blaufuks (2010a) explains how in 1941 the Nazis began using Theresienstadt fortress in occupied Czechoslovakia as a ghetto for Jews who were to be deported to the death camps in the East. In 1942 the ghetto, which had been designed to house 7000 people, had over 50,000 inmates. Starvation and illness caused over 100 deaths a day. In preparation for a visit from the International Red Cross in 1944, the city was renovated and thousands of prisoners were transferred to other camps. A community center, children's nursery, post office, bank, gymnasium, library, theater, concert hall, synagogue, and coffee shop were established. The Red Cross workers were deceived by what they saw and, encouraged by the success of their deception, the SS decided to make a fake documentary film showing life in the camp. The film was completed in 1945 and shows the captive Jews enjoying concerts, sporting events, and other leisure activities, such as reading and walking in the sun. Kurt Gerron, the Jewish inmate who directed the film, was subsequently sent to Auschwitz. All those who were forced to appear in the film were also murdered in the death camps.

Blaufuks describes first encountering a photograph of the Theresienstadt camp—showing an office with a desk, files and a clock—reproduced in Sebald's novel *Austerlitz*. In 2001, the year in which *Austerlitz* was first published, Blaufuks also came into the possession of the diaries of an individual he calls Ernst K., covering his life as a young Jewish office worker in Berlin during the period from 1926 to 1930. After undertaking further research on Ernst K., Blaufuks discovered that he had been sent with his mother to the Theresienstadt camp in 1942. Blaufuks's interest in these diaries and the fate of Ernst K. recalls the materials and methods used by Sebald to compose his fictions: found objects, stray photographs without a full account of their original context, and research into the fate of missing or displaced persons, particularly those who suffered persecution or were murdered in the Holocaust. Blaufuks decided to repeat the experiment conducted by the fictional character in Sebald's novel: as noted at the beginning of this essay, Austerlitz has a slow-motion copy made of the Nazi Theresienstadt documentary and scrutinizes it hoping to glimpse his lost mother, who was sent from Theresienstadt to Auschwitz. Similarly, Blaufuks slows down the speed of the Nazi documentary to see whether he can find Ernst K. among the inmates. He does not say whether or not this search was successful.

Through the simplest of modifications of this film—slowing its speed and tinting it red—Blaufuks achieves an ominous, dream-like atmosphere. The inmates occupy a space bathed in red light and immersed in deep sound that recalls early experiments in electronic music. We see elderly people reading, playing cards, winding a ball of wool, attending lectures, listening to a concert, or sitting outdoors in the sun. Younger people are shown doing physical exercises, running a race, playing a game of soccer. Children are shown in hospital beds, eating bread, and singing in a concert. Craftsmen and artists, tailors and seamstresses, appear in their workshops and studios, while another man slowly hammers a nail. Blaufuks's film is not silent but, because the slow speed distorts the original soundtrack, it is non-verbal. The original voice-over commentary that relays false information about the camps is now disabled. In the novel the narrator describes this effect:

At this point on that tape all that could be made out, Austerlitz continued, was a menacing growl such as I had heard only once before in my life, on an unseasonably hot May Day many years ago in the Jardin des Plantes in Paris when, after one of the peculiar turns that came over me in those days, I rested for a while on a park bench beside an aviary not far from the big cat's house, where the lions and tigers, invisible from my vantage point and, as it struck me at the time, said Austerlitz, driven out of their minds in captivity, raised their hollow roars of lament hour after hour without ceasing. (Sebald 2001, p. 250)

The official language of the Nazi bureaucracy, spoken in "high-pitched, strenuous tones" (p. 250) is revealed as a tormented, bestial howl expressing a kind of primal anxiety and terror. The violence behind the Nazi discourse of freedom through work is embodied in this deep, unsettling sound that could be aligned with the pre-verbal state of infancy. In a psychoanalytic sense, this would fit Sebald's fictional device of depicting Jacques Austerlitz searching in the film for his lost mother. The slow-motion version of the film enhances both its sinister intent and the terrible pathos of knowing that the inhabitants of the camp, going about their daily business, are all destined for destruction. It is as if the slow speed, rather than allowing the viewer to recover a lost memory, can only extend the moment before the inescapable arrival of catastrophe.

3. Trauma and Postmemory

Blaufuks's modification of the Theresienstadt film creates an immersive experience of this audiovisual archive. Despite Blaufuks's overt identification with the Holocaust victims who appear in this film, however, the question of traumatic transmission remains ambiguous. Blaufuks's use of Sebaldian strategies, including chance encounters and modification of archival materials, appears to suspend the distinction between life and death without any ultimate revelation of historical truth. This puts into question Marianne Hirsch's theory of postmemory, which has guided some interpretations of Sebald.[2] In her essay "Surviving Images: Holocaust Photographs and the Work of Postmemory," Hirsch defines postmemory as "retrospective witnessing by adoption": "It is a question of adopting the traumatic memories—and thus also the memories—of others as experiences one might oneself have had; and of inscribing them into one's own life story" (Hirsch 2001, p. 10). In her book *The Generation of Postmemory* Hirsch argues that postmemory "approximates memory in its affective force and its psychic effects" (Hirsch 2012, p. 31) and is a specifically "*generational* structure of transmission embedded in multiple forms of mediation" (Hirsch 2012, p. 35). Hirsch's account of postmemory appears to usefully describe Blaufuks's *Terezin* and Neumann's film *Austerlitz*. In both cases the filmmakers are children of Jews who directly experienced the Holocaust. Their films attempt to, in Hirsch's words, "*reactivate and re-embody*" (Hirsch 2012, p. 33) the trauma and catastrophe experienced by their parents' generation.

Hirsch argues that *Austerlitz* "played an important role in enabling the work of postmemory of an entire generation" (Hirsch 2012, p. 40). The direct relation with Holocaust survivors, whose testimony is recorded in *Shoah* and in the Fortunoff Video Archive, is now less common and collective memory is becoming more dependent on archival documents. In this situation postmemory is "shaped more and more by affect, need, and desire and time and distance attenuate the links to authenticity" (Hirsch 2012, p. 48). Kathy Behrendt, however, argues that despite Hirsch's claims, Sebald's work does not fit her account of postmemory. When Austerlitz watches the Theresienstadt film, Behrendt emphasizes the way he is "overwhelmed by the details of the past" (Behrendt 2013, p. 59) that prohibits any clear identification with the victim or recovery of lost memory. She concludes that Sebald "is engaged in a different project, and one that is best not subsumed under the umbrella of postmemory work" (Behrendt 2013, p. 60). Behrendt does not elaborate further on what this project entails, other

---

[2]   See for example (Long 2003).

than that it needs to be distinguished from postmemory, but the recent films that draw on Sebald's work may help us to clarify this distinction.

Austerlitz

In Stan Neumann's film of *Austerlitz* the voice of the novel's narrator is replaced by the commentary of the filmmaker. Unlike Sebald's German gentile narrator, Neumann is Jewish and his father was imprisoned in the Theresienstadt ghetto, suggesting a direct identification with Jacques Austerlitz. This identification also rests on Austerlitz as an amateur photographer and employs various optical devices to look at photographs. Austerlitz's request to view a slow-motion version of the Nazi documentary about Theresienstadt also characterizes him as a kind of filmmaker. At times this identification by the filmmaker with Austerlitz is stated directly. At one point the director's voice interjects: "The uneven cobblestones are firm beneath his feet, awaken his numbed senses and jolt his memory. Mine too. I see the same cobbles in photos of my childhood. And suddenly I see the book in an entirely new light, spawning the absurd idea that it was written just for me" (Neumann 2015).

The film is centered on the character of Austerlitz (played by Denis Lavant), who directly addresses the camera and delivers passages from the novel. Like *Patience*, the film is composed of journeys to different places featured in the novel—Antwerp, London (more specifically, Liverpool Street Station, the Great Eastern Hotel, and Greenwich), Paris (particularly the Bibliotheque Nationale, the Jardin des Plantes and the Gare d'Austerlitz), Marienbad, Trieste, Prague, Theresienstadt (but not Wales, the scene of Austerlitz's childhood)—and employs a Sebaldian aesthetic focusing on still photographs (some of them taken directly from the novel) but also including archival footage to give historical context, for example, the sequence that narrates the story of the German occupation of Czechoslovakia and portrays the progressive denial of civil rights to Jews.

The visual style of Neumann's *Austerlitz* shares much with *Patience*, although it is in color rather than black-and-white. The cinematography tends toward still frames and long takes, animated only by the wind in the trees or the slow movement of pedestrians through cityscapes. As in *Patience*, there are sequences shot from the windows of moving cars and trains. Black-and-white photographs feature prominently in close-up along with shots of the printed text of Sebald's book. As in *Terezin*, the Nazi documentary of the camp is reproduced in slow-motion, as described in Sebald's novel. Montages of still-framed images present various perspectives on buildings or landscapes. The melancholic pace and rhythms of Sebald's prose are translated into the cinematic languages of still images, slow cuts, slow motion and slow zoom.

The organizing metaphor in the film is architecture as a site of memory. The filmmaker uses architecture as a metaphor for trauma and identifies himself with this trauma: the destruction of the Jews in Europe. There are repeated images of boarded-up windows, suggesting that buildings contain secrets or traumatic memories that never see the light of day. The most poignant example of such an architectural secret in the book is the burial ground that lies beneath Liverpool Street Station and its connection with the *Kindertransport* that arrived there from Prague in 1939. This image reinforces the notion of traumatic transmission that underlies the filmmaker's obsession with the book—the sense that it holds a secret attraction that he must try to understand. The film closes with the filmmaker showing a photograph of his own father as a child in fancy dress, resembling the picture of Austerlitz as a child that appears on the cover of the book. In the filing room in the museum of the Theresienstadt ghetto the building takes on a specifically personal resonance for the filmmaker: "In March 1945 one of these cubbyholes contained my father's file: he was imprisoned here aged eighteen with his school resistance group. He alone survived. I was where the book had led me and has left me alone with the tenuous thread of my past" (Neumann 2015).

For Sebald, photography, film, architecture, and traumatic memory itself all appear as different forms of an encounter with something more archaic: the world of the dead. In the film of *Austerlitz* this return of the dead finds perhaps its strangest manifestation in the image of the stuffed squirrel seen in the window of a junk shop at Theresienstadt. This stuffed squirrel is mentioned but not shown in the novel. In the film it is linked to images of live squirrels in the park. Here the analogy suggested between animals and the spirits of the dead reminds us that Austerlitz begins in a zoo housing nocturnal animals—a nocturama: "It was some time before my eyes became used to its artificial dusk and I could make out different animals leading their sombrous lives behind the glass by the light of the pale moon" (Sebald 2001, p. 4). This description of the nocturama resonates with the later description of watching the slow-motion version of the Theresienstadt film:

> The only animal which has remained lingering in my memory is the raccoon. I watched it for a long time as it sat beside a little stream with a serious expression on its face, washing the same piece of apple over and over again, as if it hoped that all this washing, which went far beyond any reasonable thoroughness, would help it to escape the unreal world in which it had arrived, so to speak, through no fault of its own. (Sebald 2001, p. 4)

The men and women employed in the workshops now looked as if they were toiling in their sleep, so long did it take them to draw needle and thread through the air as they stitched, so heavily did their eyelids sink, so slowly did their lips move as they looked wearily up at the camera. They seemed to be hovering rather than walking, as if their feet no longer quite touched the ground. The contours of their bodies were blurred and, particularly in the scenes shot out of doors, in broad daylight, had dissolved at the edges (Sebald 2001, p. 247).

4. Conclusions

Blaufuks and Neumann appear to conform to Hirsch's account of postmemory in their use of Sebald's narratives to allow a transgenerational transmission of trauma. They both explicitly carry Sebald's narrative in *Austerlitz* toward a direct identification with the Jewish victim. However, the journeys that organize Sebald's fictions carry over into those different films in ways that also suggest movement back and forth between the worlds of the living and the dead and a suspension of linear temporality. Sebald's journeys and archival excavations go beyond the relationship between generations to blur the boundaries between the living and the dead, the human and non-human, between creatures and their environments or life worlds. Sebald never begins from the point of view of a direct identification with the victim. Rather, his narratives of historical catastrophe usually begin with chance encounters, found images, and journeys without any specific purpose or destination. These encounters and journeys take place in various sites, all of which are imagined as archival spaces where life has been captured and recorded but is now missing its original context and has thereby become enigmatic and elusive but also an ever-present dimension of human experience. Despite Blaufuks's and Neumann's direct concern with generational transmission, their films cannot be fully understood in terms of postmemory. Sebald's narratives demand that we suspend identification with the trauma of the Jewish victims of the Holocaust, or even with the human victims of the endless series of catastrophes that compose world history. In these films based on Sebald's books we never remain for long in any single community: we are always in transit.

Conflicts of Interest: The author declares no conflict of interest.

References

Anderson, Mark M. 2003. The Edge of Darkness: On W.G. Sebald. *October* 106: 102–21. [CrossRef]

Banki, Luisa. 2012. Mourning, Melancholia and Morality: W.G. Sebald's German-Jewish Narratives. In *Panic and Mourning: The Cultural Work of Trauma*. Edited by Daniela Agostinho, Elisa Antz and Catia Fereira. Berlin: De Gruyter, pp. 37–48.

Behrendt, Kathy. 2013. Hirsch, Sebald, and the Uses and Limits of Postmemory. In *The Memory Effect: The Remediation of Memory in Literature and Film*. Edited by Russell J.A. Kilbourn and Eleanory. Ontario: Wilfred Laurier University Press, pp. 51–67.

Benjamin, Walter. 2002. *Selected Writings, Volume 3, 1935–1938*. Edited by Howard Eiland and Michael W. Jennings. Cambridge: Harvard University Press.

Blaufuks, Daniel. 2010a. *Terezin*. Göttingen: Steidl.

Directed by Daniel Blaufuks. 2010b. *Terezin*.

Blaufuks, Daniel. 2012. *Works on Memory: Selected Writings and Images*. Cardiff: Fotogallery.

Caruth, Cathy. 1995a. Preface. In *Trauma: Explorations in Memory*. Edited by Cathy Caruth. Baltimore: Johns Hopkins University Press, pp. vii–ix.

Caruth, Cathy. 1995b. Introduction. In *Trauma: Explorations in Memory*. Edited by Cathy Caruth. Baltimore: Johns Hopkins University Press, pp. 3–12.

Felman, Shoshana, and Dori Laub. 1992. *Testimony: Crises of Witnessing in Literature, Psychoanalysis, and History*. New York and London: Routledge.

Frey, Mattias. 2007. Theorizing Cinema in Sebald and Sebald with Cinema. In *Searching for Sebald: Photography after W.G. Sebald*. Edited by Lise Patt. Los Angeles: Institute of Cultural Inquiry, pp. 226–41.

Directed by Grant Gee. 2012, *Patience (After Sebald)*. Santa Monica: Illuminations Films.

Hirsch, Marianne. 2001. Surviving Images: Holocaust Photographs and the Work of Postmemory. *Yale Journal of Criticism* 14: 5–37. [CrossRef]

Hirsch, Joshua. 2004. *Afterimage: Film, Trauma, and the Holocaust*. Philadelphia: Temple University Press.

Hirsch, Marianne. 2012. *The Generation of Postmemory: Writing and Visual Culture after the Holocaust*. New York: Columbia University Press.

Long, J. J. 2003. History, Narrative, and Photography in W.G. Sebald's *Die Ausgewanderten*. *Modern Language Review* 8: 117–37. [CrossRef]

Meek, Allen. 2010. *Trauma and Media: Theories, Histories and Images*. New York and London: Routledge.

Directed by Stan Neumann. 2015, *Austerlitz*. Strasbourg: ARTE France, Paris: Les Films d'IcI.

Pinchevski, Amit. 2011. Archive, Media, Trauma. In *On Media Memory: Collective Memory in a New Media Age*. Edited by Motti Neiger, Oren Meyers and Eyal Zandberg. New York: Palgrave MacMillan, pp. 253–64.

Scholz, Christian. 2007. 'But the Written Word is Not a True Document': A Conversation with W.G. Sebald on Literature and Philosophy. In *Searching for Sebald: Photography after W.G. Sebald*. Edited by Lise Patt. Los Angeles: Institute of Cultural Inquiry, pp. 104–9.

Sebald, W. G. 1996. *The Emigrants*. Translated by Michael Hulse. New York: New Directions.

Sebald, W. G. 1998. *Rings of Saturn*. Translated by Michael Hulse. New York: New Directions.

Sebald, W. G. 1999. *Vertigo*. Translated by Michael Hulse. New York: New Directions.

Sebald, W. G. 2001. *Austerlitz*. Translated by Anthea Bell. New York: Random House.

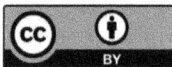

humanities

MDPI

Article

Transferential Memory Spaces in Gisela Heidenreich's *Das endlose Jahr*

Amila Becirbegovic

Department of Modern and Classical Languages and Literature, California State University, Fresno,
5245 N. Backer Ave, Fresno, CA 93740, USA; abecirbegovic@mail.fresnostate.edu; Tel.: +1-480-593-4264

Received: 23 November 2017; Accepted: 6 March 2018; Published: 15 March 2018

Abstract: What does it mean to be German after Hitler and National Socialism? Gisela Heidenreich's memoir *Das endlose Jahr: Die langsame Entdeckung der eigenen Biographie—ein Lebensborn Schicksal* (The Endless Year: The Slow Discovery of My Own Biography—A Lebensborn Destiny, 2002), highlights the dependence on physical markers and monuments in understanding one's place in history. Heidenreich discovers her origin as a Lebensborn child through family secrets, but it is not until she traverses the landscape of her past that she truly begins to understand her place within history. I argue that, along with family photographs and narratives, places play an integral role in the identity process through the metaphor of the palimpsest. In Heidenreich's memoir, the German notion of Heimat reveals itself as a process, rather than a static and immovable space. *Das endlose Jahr* addresses the interplay between memory, places, and space through Heidenreich's complex relationship with her mother, and her ambivalent sense of belonging through the palimpsest markers that remain. At its core, *Das endlose Jahr* is a memoir about the search for Heimat in all the wrong places.

Keywords: Heimat; Generationsroman; memory; space; Lebensborn; Holocaust; palimpsest; heterotopia

---

> Meine Erinnerungen haben mich
>
> heimgesucht.
>
> My memories have haunted me—*Das endlose Jahr*
>
> "Theory has shown that no space disappears completely . . . something always survives or
>
> endures."—Henri Lefebvre (1991), *The Production of Space*

In his 1969 essay, Adorno famously scrutinizes the question "What is German?", rejecting a presupposed and simplistic notion of "Germanness" (Adorno and Levin 1985, p. 121)[1]. This question, though at first glance simplistic in its formulation, encapsulates a key investigation in a contentious debate that has been raging in Germany since the end of WWII. Specifically, what does it mean to be German after Hitler and National Socialism? Being proud to be a German was deeply problematic because of the signification of Heimat, or homeland, during the Third Reich.[2] In the 19th century, Heimat developed as a strong regional identity marker. During the German Romanticist movement, Heimat became associated with typical rural life and idyllic landscapes, with an emphasis on a strong emotional investment in the places of home. As Elizabeth Boa and Rachel Palfreyman point out in *Heimat A German Dream: Regional Loyalties and National Identity in German Culture 1890–1900*,

---

[1] See Theodor Adorno's 1969 essay *On the Question "What is German?"*
[2] The German word "Heimat" has many complex significations, ranging from home to homeland, motherland, fatherland, native land, landscape, and even local history. The meaning of "Heimat" also changes regionally and nationally. Since there is no single catch-all English equivalent, I have chosen to use the German word.

the unification of Germany in 1871, as well as the Industrial Revolution, brought with it an intense paranoia and fear of a mass exodus from rural areas within Germany to more urban landscapes, dividing German identity between regional and national identity, as well as rural and urban identity (Boa and Palfreyman 2011, p. 1). Heimat thus developed as an idea of emotional attachment to home, and grew out of this fear of abandonment. The National Socialists utilized this idea of attachment to soil to further their racist rhetoric, from *Blut und Boden* (Blood and Soil) to *Lebensraum* (Living Space). Heimat became a call to action associated with racial ideologies of purity, and anyone who fell outside of the fascist ideal of a "racially pure" national identity was deemed as a threat to the National Socialist regime.

As a reaction to the fascist appropriation of the romanticist ideal of Heimat, national identity was reevaluated as a depoliticized marker of identity. From 1945–1965 Heimat was seen as an extension of nostalgia; a longing for a simpler time. Thus, Heimat became backwards-looking, focusing on rural life prior to both WWI and WWII. With a renewed interest in the memory of the Holocaust and WWII through widely publicized events, such as the Eichmann Trial (1960) and the NBC Holocaust miniseries (1978), as well as the Student movement of 1968, the question "What is German?" began to be investigated anew. The strangeness of being German in the postwar period led many to question their sense of home and to distance themselves from the previously racially laden or depoliticized definition of Heimat. In the decades since the war, arguments about German national identity have oscillated between vehement national identification and apathetic disavowal. Heimat evolved into a liminal space and a critical threshold for contemporary generations. As the decades passed, younger generations began to pursue the question "What is German?" by investigating silences. The National Socialist past was talked about in the public sphere, but not necessarily investigated in the private realm. What does it meant to be a German when your grandparents and parents were part of the Nazi regime? The *Nachgeborenen*, the postwar generation, began to grapple with their national identity. This generation felt an immense responsibility: the burden to bear witness to the crimes of the past from the vantage point of the contemporary landscape.

Gisela Heidenreich's memoir, *Das endlose Jahr: Die langsame Entdeckung der eigenen Biographie—ein Lebensborn Schicksal* (The Endless Year: The Slow Discovery of My Own Biography—A Lebensborn Destiny, 2002), approaches Germany's past through the contemporary landscape. Heidenreich demonstrates how the present remains riddled with places, markers, objects, and reminders of the Nazi past. She investigates her own mother's troubled past through the sites, places and images left behind by her family. The very soil that Heidenreich traverses is imbued with a complex postwar memory, with different generational sediments and signifiers. The old remains layered on top of the new and although buildings were rebuilt and objects reappropriated, the palimpsestic traces of the past remain legible in the present.

1. The Genealogy of Place: Founding Heimat in the *Generationsroman*

In my reading of *Das endlose Jahr*, I analyze Heimat as more than solely an emotional experience and a backward-looking model. Instead, Heimat can be understood as an extension of nostalgia, or more specifically, nostalgia for a certain place and time, which can manifest itself as forward-looking. In *The Future of Nostalgia*, Svetlana Boym emphasizes that nostalgia is longing for a home that no longer exists, or perhaps has never existed at all (Boym 2001, p. 2). Boym continues by pointing out that we often associate nostalgia with a longing for a placem when it really also is a longing for a different time (Boym 2001, p. 4). Nostalgia is the process of revisiting a specific time in history from the vantage point of the present. As Boym notes, nostalgia is therefore both retrospective, as well as prospective (Boym 2001, p. 6). By searching through the palimpsestic traces that remain in our contemporary landscape, we rediscover something about the past, but we also gather information about our present and establish a framework for how a certain event from the past will be remembered in the future. In *Excavation and Memory*, Walter Benjamin notes that "he who seeks to approach his own buried past must conduct himself like a man digging" (Benjamin et al. 2005, p. 576).[3] Those who seek to shape the future, understand their present, and experience history, must dig deep within the trenches of the past. In *Das endlose Jahr* the past is a buried image, a layering of multiple parts that must be excavated from the soil to create a whole.

Heidenreich's memoir can be characterized as part of the more contemporary network of *Familien- und Generationsromane* (family and generation novels), precisely because it features multiple generations, retelling the experiences of grandparents, parents, and their children, as they dig deep into the family archives to uncover and come to terms with the Nazi past.[4] Elisabeth Krimmer characterizes family novels as a "highly popular contemporary genre that tells 'big history' in the form of family history" often amalgamating fact and fiction (Krimmer 2015, p. 38). In *Geschichte im Gedächtnis*, Aleida Assmann makes clear that *Generationsromane* seek to reassure the character's "identity vis-à-vis her own family [as well as through] German history" (Assmann 2007, p. 73).

Heidenreich pieces her sense of self back together through the fragmented memories of family narratives. As Susan Luhmann attests, *Generationsromane* seek to "establish the extent of a family member's guilt, but also to show the continued denial of such guilt within their families" (Luhmann 2009, p. 176). Heidenreich struggles with her own sense of guilt, precisely because of her families' implication with the Nazi regime, and sets out on a quest to retrace the steps of her past.

In an effort to uncover that past, Heidenreich probes family stories, as well as official history, and emphasizes the unreliable nature of memory by exploring the dichotomy between the private and the public, focusing on uncovering the past by contrasting personal memories with official collective memory. Akin to Ruth Klüger's 1992 memoir *weiter leben: Eine Jugend* (Still Alive: A Holocaust Girlhood Remembered), *Das endlose Jahr* problematizes memory and presents it as fragmented, and at times, inaccessible. Heidenreich relies on history and family memory to reconstruct the past. However, it is only through Heidenreich's deep longing for Heimat, her nostalgia for a place and time, that those memories are affectively made real.[5] At the same time, Heidenreich acknowledges the futile desire to capture the past by reanimating places and objects to awaken memories. Similarly, Klüger contends that the desire to memorialize the past in specific sites is generally ineffective, since the essence of timescape cannot be captured, due to the "missing ingredients [such as] the odor of fear … the concentrated aggression, the reduced minds" (Klüger 1994, p. 67).[6] The palimpsestic traces of history are tangible only insofar as they are tied to a sense of *Örtlichkeit* (place). Klüger cautions that you can never truly exhume the essence of a timescape, nor should you strive to. In fact, the essence of *Örtlichkeit* may be the closest that we can come to an "authentic" memory experience. Like Klüger, Heidenreich acknowledges that these place markers are necessary bridges that connect us, however imperfectly, to times past. *Örtlichkeit* and history intricately intermingle, allowing the past to intrude on the contemporary. *Zeitschaft* (timescape) is something that remains sacred and inaccessible after time has passed, while *Örtlichkeit* offers a window into the past.

In *Generationsromane* "the discursive, social, and political frameworks of the present leave their imprint on individual recollections of the past" (Krimmer 2015, p. 38). Thus, present discourses and institutions influence the perception of the past, resulting in a memory that is often reshaped by the sites and objects deemed to be historically relevant. In his introduction to *Between Memory and History*,

---

[3]   See Alexander Kluge's 1979 film, *Die Patriotin* (The Patriotic Woman). In the film, a patriotic math teacher, Gabi Teichert, literally digs in the soil, where she discovers a dead soldier killed at the Battle of Leningrad. Through the act of digging, she is further motivated to survey the landscape, in an attempt to piece together history.

[4]   See Uwe Timm's *Am Beispiel meines Bruders* (In My Brother's Shadow, 2003), Katrin Himmler's Die Brüder Himmler: Eine deutsche Familiengeschichte (The Himmler Brothers: A German Family History, 2005), Margret Nissen's *Sind Sie die Tochter Speer?* (Are you the Daughter Speer?, 2005) and Alexander Senfft's *Schweigen tut weh: Eine deutsche Familiengeschichte* (Silence Hurts: A German Family History, 2007).

[5]   Memory and nostalgia are interlinked. Nostalgia is the longing for a different time and place, whereas memory is the recollection of that time.

[6]   For Klüger, this futile reanimation of specific sites of the past is in direct relation to her own experience as a Holocaust survivor, and her connection with the timescape of a place is solely in relation to the concentration camps.

Pierre Nora (1989) discusses the importance of *lieux de mémoire*, or sites of memory, which anchor the collective conscience of a social group. In the immediate post-WWII period, recollections of the war were inundated with fresh memory sites, evoking the recent past. *Das endlose Jahr* problematizes space through an ultimately futile search for an originary past.

2. Mothers and Daughters: The Otherness of Being Born

"Welcome home . . . you look Norwegian" (Heidenreich 2002, p. 16). The stranger warmly greets Gisela Heidenreich as she waits at a bus stop in Hønefoss, Norway, with her German mother in tow. Upon discovering that the women are in search of Gisela's birthplace in Klekken, the Norwegian man immediately offers to help drive them to the birth site, an old Norwegian hotel that was once occupied by the Nazis.[7] Since her birth, Gisela has had a distant relationship with her mother, and felt no right to a home, proclaiming that "durch meine Geburt im mit Gewalt besetzten Land habe ich mir kein 'Heimrecht' erworben" [Through my birth in a land occupied by force I have not earned a right to a home] (Heidenreich 2002, p. 22). She has always yearned to feel at home, and in an attempt to reconstruct her sense of belonging, Gisela organizes a trip with her elderly mother to visit her birthplace in Klekken.

In *Generationsromane*, growing up is often complicated by the outbreak of the war. In Heidenreich's case, this is even further problematized through her birthplace. Gisela Heidenreich was born at a Lebensborn facility in 1943 in Klekken, during the German occupation of Norway. As Patrizia Albanese outlines in *Mothers of the Nation: Women, Families and Nationalism in 20th Century Europe*, the Lebensborn e.V., or Lebensborn (fount of life) registered association was initiated by the SS and formed in 1935 (Albanese 2006, pp. 37–38). The association sought to raise the birthrate of Aryan children, who were to become the future soldiers and leaders of Germany. The association accomplished this by providing welfare to unmarried, or single German women during their pregnancy. In addition to services provided to women and SS members, it was discovered at the Nuremberg Trials that these facilities often engaged in the transfer of children, mostly orphans, or children kidnapped from Eastern Europe, to families in Germany. The association encouraged and mediated the adoption of children born on site or brought to the Lebensborn facility. As the war progressed, Lebensborn expanded into several occupied European countries with Germanic populations, most prominently in Poland, Denmark, and Norway. Heidenreich's unwed German mother was transferred to work at the Lebensborn facility from her job as a secretary for the SS-Junkerschule Bad Tölz, an officer's training school for the Waffen-SS. After her romantic relationship with a prominent married SS officer, Heidenreich's mother was transported to the Norwegian facility, where she gave birth to Gisela.

Akin to other Lebensborn children, such as Ann-Frid Lyngstad, Heidenreich's origin story propels her on a quest to get to know her "real" Heimat. Gisela Heidenreich's mother, Emilie Edelmann, a very composed, stern, and unsentimental woman, often left young Gisela in need of affection. As a child, because of her Lebensborn origin, her biological mother initially disowned her and Gisela was raised by her aunt, whom she referred to as her mother for the first formative years of her life. Later, Gisela's mother revealed herself to be her real mother, leaving young Gisela confused and rejected. Gisela recalls how her mother would often cross the road abruptly if she saw someone on the sidewalk from the Junkerschule, or even an old neighbor, or friend. Her mother would let go of Gisela's hand, leaving her alone on the other side of the street, so as not to rouse suspicion that Gisela was her child (Heidenreich 2002, p. 115). Gisela was never allowed to feel at home, not even in the presence of her mother.

---

[7] In *Das endlose Jahr*, Gisela's mother Emilie Edelmann does not recognize the hotel as the old Lebensborn location, either intentionally, as a way to avoid confronting the Nazi past in the present landscape, or simply because the hotel does not look like it did many decades ago. Instead, Emilie claims that a school several miles from the hotel was the actual Lebensborn site. Gisela discovers, however, that the hotel, which the mother was quick to dismiss as the wrong site, was the actual Lebensborn location.

Deprived of both nation and maternal affection, Gisela feels *heimatlos* (homeless), a condition that manifests itself as a perpetual feeling of otherness. Whenever Gisela felt secure and at home in her surroundings and in her relationship with her mother, the rug was pulled from under her. The spaces that were supposed to be familiar—the street, the school, and even the home—became spaces of otherness, ultimately becoming what Michel Foucault, in a 1967 lecture to an audience of architects titled "Of Other Spaces", terms heterotopias. Foucault posits that spaces are formed through society, and rely on social structures of power. However, when the social order is inverted, a disturbance of place occurs (Foucault and Rabinow 2010, p. 24). Heterotopias are parallel spaces, exemplifying otherness. They are counter-sites and places that are only able to exist in relation to other places, containing the undesirable, in order to make space for the envisioned notion of a utopia elsewhere. They exhibit many layers of meaning in relation to other places. Foucault outlines that heterotopic spaces are transitory spaces where adolescents, pregnant women, or the elderly come to live out a fleeting moment in their lives (Foucault and Rabinow 2010, p. 5). Thus, the Lebensborn facility in Norway is a kind of crisis heterotopia, where Gisela comes into the world, but is hidden away in a parallel space. Gisela's existence is therefore riddled with contradictions, a characteristic inherent in heterotopias of deviation. Her world is representative of many dualities, from her struggle between her home in Germany and her birthplace in Norway, to her relationship with her mother.

Heterotopias capture moments that shape how one ultimately sees oneself in relation to the other. Gisela's mother is a disturbance to Gisela's process of self-identification, acting as the ultimate stranger, embodying a space that should be familiar, but ultimately becomes *unheimlich* (uncanny). To invoke Sigmund Freud's *Das Unheimliche* (The Uncanny), what is *heimlich* becomes *unheimlich*, precisely because the unfamiliar is initially domestically familiar (Freud and Gay 1999, pp. 577–81). Simple everyday objects, and even familiar people, feelings, and experiences can suddenly become alien. Thus, the uncanny is something that is strangely familiar, as embodied by the subject's own simultaneous attraction and repulsion towards the uncanny subject. When we look at Gisela's relationship with her mother, she is at once the daughter and the hidden, secret Other in the family. Her fractured relationship with her family repeatedly drives her into confrontations with uncanny spaces. As someone without a home, without a mother, and someone who cannot assimilate into the spaces around her, Gisela sees herself as the other. As this other Gisela occupies a space comparable to the Foucauldian heterotopia, insofar as a heterotopic space also questions and subverts the logic governing social functions and relations. The disturbance brought on through the strained mother–daughter relationship creates parallel spaces bearing elements of the heterotopic, from which Gisela is able to reflect on the past and challenge and subvert the logic and functions of the monuments, sites, and places that she encounters.

3. Das Endlose Jahr: Searching for Home in All the Wrong Places

As she stands in a Norwegian museum, the words "welcome home" echo in Gisela's head, leaving her riddled with guilt. The visit to Klekken was meant as a reconciliation trip between mother and daughter. Emilie's demeanor as a mother is complicated through her role in the opening of the first Lebensborn facility in Klekken, Norway in 1941. Emilie never shared the details of her troubled past with her daughter, and Gisela learned about Lebensborn only by stumbling upon the salacious reporting of Will Berthold in his fictitious journalistic essays about the "secrets of the Lebensborn houses", and later, in his 1958 novel, *Lebensborn e.V. Ein Tatsachenroman* (Lebensborn registered association: A non-fictional novel). Even during this reconciliation trip in Norway, Emilie often conceals the truth, declining to recall and recount certain facts, locations and instances, eventually outright refusing to even visit many of the sites that hint at the Nazi past in Norway. Gisela treks through Oslo alone, visiting museums and monuments, hoping to fill the gaps in her own biography, yet again, without the help of her mother. At a museum exhibit about the Anti-Nazi resistance in Oslo, Gisela stops dead in her tracks. The sign above the exhibit reads "1943—Et Langt Ar—The Endless Year" (Heidenreich 2002, p. 33).[8] The exhibit depicts the Nazi occupation of Norway and Hitler's secret command to overtake the Scandinavian countries. By 9 April 1940 Norway was attacked and occupied in a *Nacht und Nebel* (Night and Fog) action. Gisela cannot muster the courage to keep going, and is afraid of the pain that her birth year has caused for the many families and citizens of Norway. Nevertheless, she pushes on and discovers a jarring display of monuments and photographs of Norwegian citizens who suffered under the occupation of the Nazis.

At its core, *Das endlose Jahr* is a memoir about the search for Heimat in all the wrong places. As Ruth Klüger recognizes in *weiter leben,* "to conjure up the dead you have to dangle the bait of the present before them, the flesh of the living, [in order] to coax them out of their inertia" (Klüger 2001, p. 69). The search for places that capture the past and "awaken the dead" are repeatedly intertwined with the task of "returning" home. Gisela must return to the place of her birth in an attempt to piece together the past. The digging up of history and excavation of memory can only be carried out in the shifting ground of the present. For Gisela, sites of memory haunt the present landscape and, through them, she is able to forge a bridge between the dead and the living.

Gisela returns again and again to her birthplace, wandering the streets of her uncanny Heimat, recognizing that we cannot evoke the physical reality of the past, and are forever bound to lose the essence of *Zeitschaft.* However, the *Örtlichkeit* can be restored through images, objects, and structures, which bring alive a synthetic *Zeitschaft.* In other words, though the recreation of the timescape is artificial, as the essence of time cannot be recaptured, the experience is affectively charged, so as to seem real. Gisela has no personal memories of her hometown, and must artificially reconstruct the past.

In *Berlin Childhood around 1900,* Walter Benjamin comments on memory and the traces the past leaves behind, noting that photographs can awaken a strong sense of homesickness (Benjamin et al. 2005, p. 37). Imagery, in general, holds the potential for a powerful affective recall, by introducing a longing for the past and nostalgia for Heimat through visual cues. Images provide an entry point into the past, signaling and reminding the viewer what once was. By relying on recognition through nostalgic cues, such as people and experiences, the image establishes an affective link, bridging the past and present. As David Altheide notes in his analysis of journalism and media, *how* certain images and information are presented to us as a society determines *what* we believe, in turn shaping our perception of our identity (Altheide 2002, pp. 42–44).[9] Images can be geared towards an element of nostalgic voyeurism (Altheide 2002, p. 41). According to Altheide, the viewer feels as if she is witnessing the events through the simulation of a familiar space, often relying on a physical landmark, which animates the imagery of the event in the imagination of the audience (Altheide 2002, p. 31). Thus, memory is dependent not solely on images, but also on objects and physical sites to capture the attention of the audience and to bring alive the events of the past. These sites, which I refer to as "palimpsest markers", bring the past alive through recycled and recognizable formats, from specific structures and buildings, to cities, countries and locations more generally. Through palimpsest markers we are able to see traces of the past in the present landscape. Similar to palimpsest manuscripts and architecture, the past has been reused and scraped off to make room for new texts, images and structures. What matters is not what form these palimpsest markers take on, rather, that they encapsulate a feeling of the past and an affective link to history through nostalgia.

When we enter a space, it conjures certain thoughts, and through these thoughts, the spaces become connected to other imagery places. This is how we form and mix memories, allowing the

---

[8] In Heidenreich's memoir, the Norwegian (Et Langt Ar) and English (The Endless Year) appear side by side as a direct translation from the museum exhibit. A more straightforward translation of "et langt år" would simply be "a long year/ein langes Jahr".

[9] Emphasis added.

past and present to intersect and collide. Though initially satisfied and emotionally affected by the places, images and things that she absorbed at the Norwegian museum and at her birth site, Gisela still does not *feel* at home. The burden of the past weighs heavily on her, but none of the places in and around Oslo have provided that affective bridge between the past and the present that Gisela seeks, leaving her *heimatlos* (homeless) once again. Unable to relate to her surroundings in Germany and to her "new home" in Norway, she feels disappointed that this trip did not provide her with all of the answers that she was looking for. On her last day before returning to Germany, Gisela decides to take in one last tourist attraction, seemingly unrelated to the war. In an attempt to clear her head, she decides to visit the gigantic Frogner Park, an eighty acre park in the city center of Oslo, housing the Vigeland installation, a project of 212 bronze and granite sculptures designed by the famous Norwegian artist Gustav Vigeland. Gisela's mother declines to come along once again, claiming that "de Nackerten muss ich mir net noch einmal anschau'n" [I don't have to look at the naked people again] (Heidenreich 2002, p. 69).

The sculptures depict naked men, women, and babies, designed to represent the evolution of human life from birth to death. As Gisela approaches Vigeland's sculpture of a mother twirling her young child, she is reminded of a personal photograph. Emilie Edelmann proudly displayed family photos in an album. As a young child, Gisela often searched through this album, looking for photographs of herself, but she never found any. It was not until Gisela discovered a hidden box, labeled "Gisi," tucked away in a closet, that she saw her first baby pictures (Heidenreich 2002, p. 192).

The photographs are somber mementos, depicting a stern Emilie and a sad looking blond and blue eyed young Gisela. The only image that captures a moment of genuine happiness is a photo of Emilie proudly twirling an infant Gisela in front of her sister's house in southern Germany.

As Roland Barthes notes in *Camera Lucida*, photography is a medium uniquely in touch with loss, and captures a sentiment as certain as remembrance (Barthes 2010, p. 70). In other words, photographs have a haunting power to involuntarily creep back up in the viewer at a later time, invoking a memory of the past and capturing a certain affective sentiment of the photographic subject for the viewer. In Barthes's theory of photographic representation, the image retains what he calls an "umbilical" connection to its referent. The photograph attests that what one sees has indeed existed in the past (Barthes 2010, p. 82), providing an entry point into history. It is not surprising, then, that Gisela has a strong emotional response to this particular image evoking a maternal moment between mother and child. However, Gisela only recalls this photograph in response to the Vigeland sculpture depicting a similar image of a mother twirling her infant.

Gisela's first impulse is to recoil at the sight of the naked figures. She reflects, "ich bin nicht besonders begeistert von den naturalistischen Darstellungen fast makelloser Körper, zu sehr erinnern sie mich tatsächlich an Naziskulpturen und die Kunst des sozialistischen Realismus" [I am not thrilled with the naturalistic representations of nearly flawless bodies. They remind me too much of the Nazi sculptures and the art associated with socialist realism] (Heidenreich 2002, p. 70). The sculptures evoke various associations for Gisela, reminding her initially of the many sculptures that Hitler commissioned during the Third Reich. In his essay "Nazi Aesthetics", Carsten Strathausen focuses on the function of Nazi art, highlighting its aim to depict a romanticized view of reality, an idealized image (Strathausen 2004, p. 8). The real was transformed into the realm of ideas, through the elevation of one image, usually the representation of the flawless, strong, and often masculine body, as a symbol of the fascist model of nation, health and strength (Strathausen 2004, p. 8). Here, however, the symbolic image is the antithesis of the Nazi idealized male body. The focus is instead on the mother–child relationship, as an extension of motherland/Heimat, forcing Gisela to confront her own troubled past through her relationship with her mother.

Gisela quickly moves from discomfort to being deeply moved. She notices the similarities between the Vigeland sculptures and her own experience as a mother.

> Dennoch rühren sie mich an, manche Szenen wirken tatsächlich wie dem Leben nachgestellt
> ... Eine Figur zieht mich besonders an: Eine junge Frau hebt ein Baby mit ausgestreckten

Armen hoch...Ich fotografiere die Plastik von allen Seiten, die Szene ist mir vertraut: Ich erinnere mich, wie ich meine Kinder, als sie so klein waren, ähnlich glücklich durch die Luft wirbelte und wie sie glucksten vor Vergnügen. Warum denn werde ich traurig, werden meine Augen schon wieder feucht?

[Nevertheless they affect me, some scenes even appear to be lifelike ... one figure in particular draws me in: A young woman lifts her baby with outstretched arms ... I photograph the figure from all sides, the scene is familiar: I remember, when my children were little, how I twirled them through the air as they gurgled with joy. Why then do I become sad and why do my eyes begin to water?] (Heidenreich 2002, p. 70).

According to Barthes, a photograph "is never distinguished from its referent (Barthes 2010, p. 5), and this moment of identification, between sculpture and real-life experience as mediated through a photograph, is integral in animating and triggering Gisela's affective response to the image of her and her mother, moving her to tears. As Marianne Hirsch (1997) points out in *Family Frames: Photography, Narrative and Postmemory*, photographs have a strong affective power in connecting generations. Hirsch outlines the relationship that the generation after bears to the traumatic memory of those who came before. Hirsch's term, postmemory, focuses on the power of images to signal to the viewer what the past looked like and provides an essential affective link and an edge of specificity. Postmemory can best be described as a haunting intruder, a spectral memory that unexpectedly reintroduces the past in the present. According to Hirsch, images can become historical access points that allow the second generation to understand the context of the historical events. It is precisely the connection between photograph and life that triggers Gisela's memory of her past. Barthes notes that "a specific photograph reaches me; it animates me, and I animate it" (Barthes 2010, p. 20). Certain photographs then possess a strong affective attraction between referent and viewer, evoking "tiny jubilations" (Barthes 2010, p. 16) within the observer.

This kind of emotional connection to her past is what Gisela was desperately searching for through family narratives. Regardless of the bits and pieces of information that she was able to gather in the process of investigating her past, she always felt distant and removed from this history, unable to truly connect. What was missing was an affective link, a space that would bring the past emotionally alive again in the present. As Alison Landsberg notes in *Prosthetic Memory*, a transferential space is vital in bringing the past into a thinkable and palatable context for the present (Landsberg 2004, pp. 120–21). Transferential spaces are aptly named because they transfer memories affectively. Gisela's affective response to the Vigeland mother and child sculpture is triggered by her own familial connection to history through her mother. Thus, Gisela's identification process with the sculptures works twofold. First, she is able to relate to the monument because of her own experiences as a mother and also, in part, because of her complex history with her own mother. Secondly, Gisela is able to relate to history through imagery that is also unrelated to her own personal history. It was not until Gisela stood at Frogner Park in Norway that she was able to experience that affective connection to history, bridging an important emotional gap between the past and the present. See Figures 1 and 2.

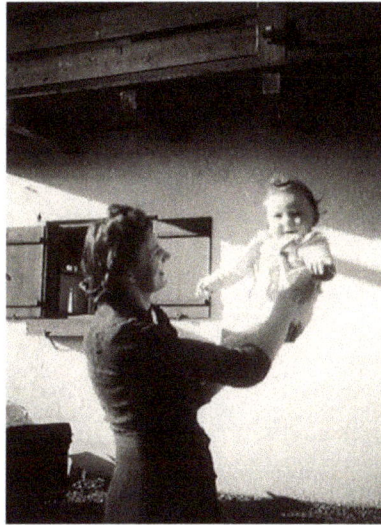

Figure 1. Gisela Heidenreich as a baby with her mother, Emilie Edelmann.

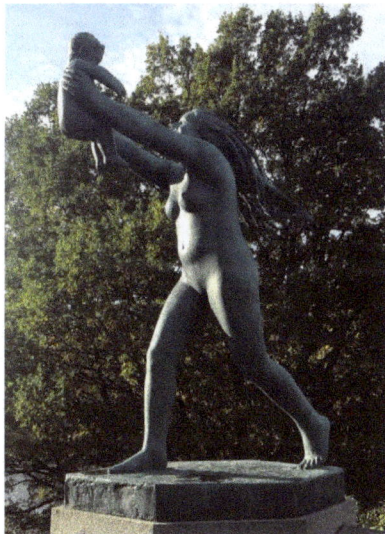

Figure 2. *Mother and Child* by Gustav Vigeland, Vigeland Sculpture Park inside Frogner Park in Oslo, Norway ©Amila Becirbegovic.

The most popular attraction sits at the highest point in Frogner Park. Gisela finally arrives at the wrought iron gates that take on the form of human bodies. She has finally come face to face with the forty-six-foot high monolith, made up of 121 human figures rising towards the sky, carved from a single piece of granite. The monolith is designed to represent man's desire to commune with the spiritual world. The humans embracing each other are carved as if they are being carried towards salvation, propelled upwards together. Work on the structure began in 1924, and was finally unveiled in 1944, a year after Gisela's birth.

Gisela is struck by the sheer size of the sculpture, but also by its resemblance to images from the concentration camps. She recalls "auch wenn diese glatt und wohlgenährt sind und die Skulptur die Form eines riesigen Phallus hat, erinnert sie mich an die Fotos von den Leichenbergen in den Konzentrationslagern" [Even if the figures are flat and well fed and the sculpture is in the form of a giant phallus, I am still reminded of the photos of mass graves in the concentration camps] (Heidenreich 2002, p. 75). Though Vigeland could not have predicted the resemblance between his "human pillar" and the images of the mass graves and bodies being bulldozed during the liberation of the camps, his intertwined bodies provide a transferential space to catapult Gisela into a moment in history that she herself did not experience. See Figure 3.

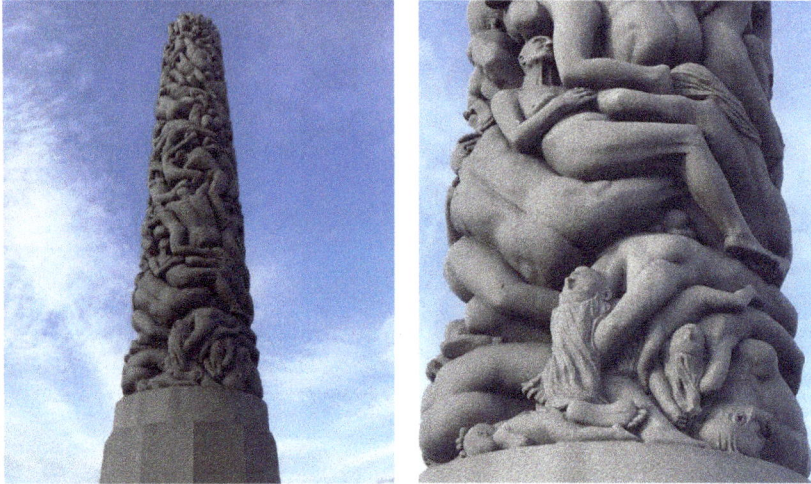

Figure 3. Forty-six-foot high monolith by Gustav Vigeland with 121 human figures. Vigeland Sculpture Park inside Frogner Park in Oslo, Norway ©Amila Becirbegovic.

In accordance with Gary Weissman's argument in *Fantasies of Witnessing*, Gisela *feels* the need to witness the past as if she were there, to study, remember, and memorialize the Holocaust and the atrocities committed by the Nazis (Weissman 2004, p. 4). Weissman describes this process of *feeling* and visualizing the Holocaust as a "fantasy of witnessing", and highlights the desire of those who did not live through the event to experience the past, whether through museums, monuments, images, or films (Weissman 2004, p. 15). Weissmann theorizes this process as a desire to act as a witness to the past. However, as Weissman makes clear, we are not witnessing the actual events of the Holocaust, but instead "experiencing representations of the Holocaust" (Weissman 2004, p. 20). Whereas firsthand accounts and "family connections grant children of survivors a 'position of privilege' closer, as it were, to the Holocaust" (Weissman 2004, p. 21), non-witnesses must work to construct a different space in relation to the event. Thus, Gisela constructs this space for herself through images, which she is vividly reminded of by Vigeland's monolith. This phenomenon of reconstructing memory through palimpsest markers and objects is often achieved by recalling the most horror-filled and iconic imagery from the past. In Gisela's case, though she does not explicitly identify the images by name, she invokes the widely publicized photos of the mass graves from April of 1945, during the liberation of concentration camp Bergen-Belsen.[10] However anachronistically, the human pillar strongly *seems* to

---

[10] Many of these images depicting mass graves are in fact taken as part of the "clean-up" effort of the British forces who were trying to get decomposing bodies buried quickly to prevent the spread of disease.

reference one shot in particular, depicting Dr. Fritz Klein, a Nazi physician tried for his crimes at the Belsen Trials and subsequently hung, standing on a heap of mangled bodies. Much like Vigeland's monolith, the grey bodies are piled up so high in the Klein photograph that they reach out of the frame, suggesting an endless cascade of corpses. It is no surprise that Gisela is able to call up this memory of the camps when confronted with the gigantic Vigeland sculpture. She herself recalls later in the narrative how, upon watching a film about the liberation of the camps at school, she could not shake the images from her memory. "Nie mehr habe ich die Bilder der lebenden Skelette in den gestreiften Anzügen, in zerschlissene Decken gehüllt, die sich gegenseitig stützen, vergessen . . . Die Leichenberge. Die Brillen. Die Kleider-und Haarhaufen" [I have never forgotten the images of the living skeletons in striped uniforms, who were enveloped in blankets as they held each other up . . . the mass graves. The glasses. The heaps of clothes and hair] (Heidenreich 2002, p. 160).

4. Conclusions: Transferential Spaces in Unexpected Places

The same affective link that photographs rely on can be experienced through the awareness of a space. These palimpsest traces, still often physically present in contemporary structures, can often go unnoticed, much as an old family photo can go unnoticed tucked away in a drawer. However, physical markers, such as monuments, cannot be tucked away. The presence of spaces associated with the Nazi past unsettles the setting they occupy, and intrudes on the present landscape. Thus, palimpsest markers haunt the present with memories of the past, and evoke both feelings of nostalgia for, and dread of, Heimat. Heidenreich begins her memoir with a quote from philosopher George Santayana's *Reason in Common Sense*: "Wer sich der Vergangeheit nicht erinnert, ist verurteilt, sie erneut zu durchleben" [Those who do not remember the past are sentenced to relive/repeat it] (Santayana 1982, p. 284). *Das endlose Jahr* is most immediately a memoir about a woman's attempt to relive her past through places and spaces.

The many sites, monuments, and images that she is confronted with on her trip to Norway facilitate Gisela's insistent quest to remember and understand her past. Gisela aptly begins this search in Norway, not Germany. Her obsession with the past and insistence on retracing the steps of history become visible in her quest to find her birthplace. However, Gisela's trip to Norway is not enough to recreate a complete sense of Heimat.

Gisela returns to Bad Tölz, her childhood home in Bavaria, after suffering sudden sensorineural hearing loss and, quite literally, begins a healing process.[11] On her doctor's orders to return to Bad Tölz, where she can be surrounded by friends and family (Heidenreich 2002, p. 216), Gisela sets out on a second journey to come to terms with her past, this time in her German Heimat. She notes upon her arrival, "meine Erinnerungen haben mich heimgesucht" [My memories have haunted me] (Heidenreich 2002, p. 217). The specters of Gisela's past have driven her back to Germany in an effort to heal. She notes, "vielleicht gehört es zu meiner 'Heilung', dass ich an Ort und Stelle endgültig mit meiner Kindheit 'ins Reine' kommen kann" [Maybe it is part of my 'healing process' that I can here and now definitively come to terms with my childhood] (Heidenreich 2002, p. 217). Thus, Gisela confronts each childhood trauma, from the time her uncle tried to kill her simply for being an "SS-Bankert" (SS bastard) to the time the American soldiers burst into her aunt's house, ransacking their belongings and chasing them out of their home. Gisela approaches each trauma, each memory of her troubled past, through the various sites of her childhood, from Norway to Germany. Each new landscape and each marker awakens a vivid recollection, catapulting Gisela into the memories of her past. With time Gisela's hearing loss heals, disappearing as suddenly as it came on, and with it

---

[11] Sudden sensorineural hearing loss is not well understood, and results in an often-temporary hearing loss. It can be attributed to acoustic trauma, in response to loud sounds, or autoimmune inner ear diseases and viral infections of the inner ear. In Gisela Heidenreich's case, the first onset of her temporary hearing loss is brought on by a fight with her elderly mother after their reconciliation trip to Norway. Thus, her hearing loss can be interpreted as a psychosomatic response to her fraught relationship with her mother and her own unfinished past.

her deeply rooted anxieties of being *heimatlos*. Gisela makes peace with her former childhood home and even embarks on a journey to get to know her biological father, a married former SS officer.[12] Gisela Heidenreich's healing process tellingly began in Norway, through encounters with monuments of an unknown past. Her narrative comes full circle as she wanders the streets and sites of her former home in Germany.

Das endlose Jahr accesses memories through palimpsest markers, in an effort to integrate the past into the contemporary landscape, rather than solely coming to terms with it and settling the score. In *The Condition of Postmodernity*, David Harvey expresses the view that the modern city, or any material modern space, is like a theater, developing into a series of stages upon which individuals can perform a multiplicity of roles (Harvey 2000, p. 5). The dependence on physical markers and monuments in *Das endlose Jahr* encapsulates a kind of memory stage; in each instance, the memories of the past are relived through places. As Harvey notes, the essence of time is thus impossible to capture from a single perspective. Instead, memory is constructed from multiple perspectives (Harvey 2000, p. 30), through one memory folding into another as time progresses. As evidenced by Gisela Heidenreich's journey, discovering Heimat can come from unexpected places. Since timescape is inaccessible, Heidenreich seeks a transferential memory space through often unexpected sites. Thus, Heimat is a process, rather than a static and immovable space, changing in response to historical circumstances and individual recollections. While our identities remain tied to our sense of home and to the collective, our sense of home has become far more malleable. As Adorno points out, "Germanness" is not necessarily a simple identity marker. We strive to consolidate our understanding of history with our understanding of what it means to be at home today—a notion of home that is constantly shifting and evolving.

Conflicts of Interest: The author declares no conflict of interest.

References

Adorno, Theodor W., and Thomas Y. Levin. 1985. On the Question: 'What Is German?'. *New German Critique* 36: 121–31. [CrossRef]

Albanese, Patrizia. 2006. *Mothers of the Nation: Women, Families and Nationalism in Twentieth-Century Europe.* Toronto: University of Toronto Press.

Altheide, David L. 2002. *Creating Fear: News and the Construction of Crisis.* New York: Aldine De Gruyter.

Assmann, Aleida. 2007. *Geschichte im Gedächtnis: Von der individuellen Erfahrung zur öffentlichen Inszenierung.* Munich: C. H. Beck.

Barthes, Roland. 2010. *Camera Lucida: Reflections on Photography.* New York: Hill and Wang.

Benjamin, Walter, Michael W. Jennings, Howard Eiland, and Gary Smith. 2005. *Walter Benjamin: Selected Writings.* Cambridge: Belknap, vol. 2, Part 2.

Boa, Elizabeth, and Rachel Palfreyman. 2011. *Heimat: A German Dream: Regional Loyalties and National Identity in German Culture 1890–1990.* Oxford: Oxford University Press.

Boym, Svetlana. 2001. *The Future of Nostalgia.* New York: Basic Books.

Foucault, Michel, and Paul Rabinow. 2010. *The Foucault Reader.* New York: Vintage, Random House.

Freud, Sigmund, and Peter Gay. 1999. *The Freud Reader.* New York: Norton.

Harvey, David. 2000. *The Condition of Postmodernity.* Oxford: Blackwell.

Heidenreich, Gisela. 2002. *Das endlose Jahr: Die langsame Entdeckung der eigenen Biographie—Ein Lebensbornschicksal.* Bern: Scherz, Munich: Scherz.

Heidenreich, Gisela. 2007. *Sieben Jahre Ewigkeit: Eine deutsche Liebe.* Munich: Droemer.

Heidenreich, Gisela. 2011. *Geliebter Täter: Ein Diplomat im Dienst der "Endlösung".* Munich: Droemer.

---

12 See Gisela Heidenreich's *Sieben Jahre Ewigkeit. Eine deutsche Liebe* (Heidenreich 2007) and *Geliebter Täter. Ein Diplomat im Dienst der "Endlösung"* (Heidenreich 2011).

Hirsch, Marianne. 1997. *Family Frames: Photography, Narrative, and Postmemory*. Cambridge: Harvard University Press.

Klüger, Ruth. 1994. *weiter leben: Eine Jugend*. Munich: Deutscher Taschenbuch Verlag.

Klüger, Ruth. 2001. *Still Alive: A Holocaust Girlhood Remembered*. New York: Feminist Press.

Krimmer, Elisabeth. 2015. The Representation of Wartime Rape in Julia Franck's *Die Mittagsfrau* and Jenny Erpenbeck's *Heimsuchung*. *Gegenwartsliteratur* 14: 35–60.

Landsberg, Alison. 2004. *Prosthetic Memory: The Transformation of American Remembrance in the Age of Mass Culture*. New York: Columbia University Press.

Lefebvre, Henri. 1991. *The Production of Space*. Oxford: Blackwell.

Luhmann, Susanne. 2009. Gender and the Generations of Difficult Knowledge: Recent Responses to Familial Legacies of Nazi Perpetration. *Women in German Yearbook* 25: 174–98.

Nora, Pierre. 1989. Between Memory and History: Les Lieux de Mémoire. *Representations* 26: 7–24. [CrossRef]

Santayana, George. 1982. *Reason in Common Sense*. Mineola: Dover. First published 1929.

Strathausen, Carsten. 2004. Nazi Aesthetics. *Culture, Theory and Critique* 42: 5–19. [CrossRef]

Weissman, Gary. 2004. *Fantasies of Witnessing: Postwar Efforts to Experience the Holocaust*. Ithaca: Cornell University Press.

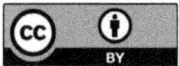

MDPI

St. Alban-Anlage 66

4052 Basel, Switzerland

Tel. +41 61 683 77 34

Fax +41 61 302 89 18

http://www.mdpi.com

Humanities Editorial Office

E-mail: humanities@mdpi.com

http://www.mdpi.com/journal/humanities

www.ingramcontent.com/pod-product-compliance
Lightning Source LLC
Chambersburg PA
CBHW051909210326
41597CB00033B/6082